Tissue Economies

SCIENCE AND CULTURAL THEORY

A Series Edited by Barbara Herrnstein Smith

and E. Roy Weintraub

A JOHN HOPE FRANKLIN CENTER BOOK

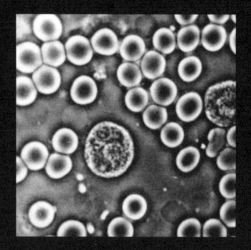

Tissue Economies

BLOOD, ORGANS, AND CELL LINES

IN LATE CAPITALISM

Catherine Waldby and Robert Mitchell

DUKE UNIVERSITY PRESS   Durham and London   2006

2nd Printing, 2007

© 2006 Duke University Press

Printed in the United States of America

on acid-free paper ∞

Designed by C. H. Westmoreland

Typeset in Scala by Keystone Typesetting, Inc.

Library of Congress Cataloging-in-Publication

Data appear on the last printed page

of this book.

Contents

Acknowledgments

Catherine Waldby would like to thank, first of all, her wonderful colleagues at Brunel University, London. In particular she wishes to acknowledge the unfailing enthusiasm and humor of Alan Irwin, and the kindness and support of Ian Robinson. Numerous friends and colleagues made intellectual life in London rich and exciting. Thanks to John Stringer and Alan Waters for the civilized pleasures of Ealing; to Celia Lury, Mariam Fraser, Marsha Rosengarten, Mike Michaels, and many other colleagues at Goldsmith's College for their incisive critiques and good company; to Nikolas Rose, Karen Throsby, Carlos Novas, and the rest of the BIOS crew for their intellectual generosity and friendship; to Nina Wakeford and Nicola Green for their sociable collaborations around feminism and technology; to Celia Roberts, Adrian McKenzie, Alan Petersen, and Roz Porter for their hospitality and our ongoing conversations about medicine, the body, and technology. Catherine also thanks Andrew Webster for his support and assistance; Donna Dickenson for her generosity with her exhaustive knowledge of tissue economies in the United Kingdom; Susan Squier for her imaginative engagement and collaborative spirit; Melinda Cooper for her extraordinary scholarship and conversation; and Susan Kippax for innumerable forms of institutional, collegial, and personal support. Lastly, Catherine thanks her partner, Paul Jones, her friends Pam Hansford and Anne Brewster, and her family—David, Valerie, Gavan, Jenny, Madison, and Sebastian—for their love and support.

Robert Mitchell wishes to thank Phillip Thurtle, who always provides invaluable responses to all questions and queries; Shannon

Callies, whose third kidney was the starting point for one of these chapters; Donald Mitchell, who has always proved an eager and willing correspondent on the past and future of capitalism; and Matt Cohen, Lauren Dame, James Boyle, Inga Pollmann, Arti Rai, Patrick and Sharon Terry, and Priscilla Wald, whose comments significantly improved several of these chapters. He also thanks the Josiah Charles Trent Memorial Foundation Grant for funds which assisted in interviews with the co-founders of PXE International, and the students who participated in the course "Cultural Narratives of Genomics" at Duke University in the fall of 2004 (and an especial thanks to the teaching assistant for that course, Erin Gentry).

We would both like to thank the organizers of, and participants in, conferences at which we presented early versions of this material, including the Society for Literature and Science conference in Denmark, 2002, where this project began; the Society for Literature and Science conference in Pasadena, California, 2002; the BIOS seminar series and the BIOS conference "Vital Politics" at the London School of Economics in 2003; the Literature and Genetics Colloquium at Vanderbilt and Duke Universities in 2003 and 2004; and the conference of the Society for Social Studies of Science/EASST in Paris, 2004. Finally, we thank the two anonymous readers of our manuscript, whose comments and suggestions greatly enriched the final version of this book, and Raphael Allen, Reynolds Smith, Courtney Berger, and all the others at Duke University Press who have made this book possible.

Introduction

Blood, Community, and September 11 Within hours of the terrorist attacks on the World Trade Center, the U.S. Department of Health and Human Services, the American Association of Blood Banks, and the American Red Cross issued calls for people to donate blood. Supplies were low throughout the state of New York. Four days before the attacks, state hospitals and health professionals had convened a meeting to discuss ways to improve the blood supply (Butler 2001). In the chaos following the attacks, health authorities could not estimate how many people were injured, or what quantities of transfusion blood they might need. Immediately thousands of people came forward to give blood. They waited in line for hours. The New York Blood Center, which supplies most of the city's hospitals, collected more than five thousand units of blood and fielded twelve thousand phone calls in the first twelve hours. In Washington, after the terrorist attack on the Pentagon, blood was collected at hospitals, makeshift centers, and a building next to the White House (Schmidt 2002). When the collection centers closed, many people queued through the night. At 6:30 the next morning there were already long lines outside blood banks (*Guardian*, 12 September 2001). Hospitals, already dealing with the wounded and dying, had difficulty finding enough trained staff to test donated blood, or storage capacity to accept the volume offered.

This overwhelming desire to give blood was not limited to the citizens of New York and Washington: all over the United States, similar scenes were played out. In the weeks following September 11, more than 475,000 units were collected for the victims, but only 258 units were used for them, and much of the blood had to be discarded (Schmidt 2002).

What was going on here? What can explain this response to a national disaster? Why did the citizens of the United States, after years of declining blood donation,[1] rush to give blood in the wake of the terrorist attack? To cast the question a little wider, what does it mean to give blood, and why does a national disaster elicit such a response? It is self-evident that for the people queuing, giving blood was a pragmatic means of helping those injured in the attack. They were acting on a model of the body, and of relationships between bodies, that we take for granted in the twenty-first century: one body can share its vitality with another through the redistribution of tissues, from donor to recipient, through biotechnical intervention. As the lucky ones, the healthy ones, they can give a portion of their blood, a self-renewing substance, to those who have lost blood in the violence of the attacks. A blood transfusion may mean the difference between living and dying. In this sense the donors give to victims a little of their health. In the face of a horrifying spectacle of death, the donors can give life.

It seems to us, however, that the desire to give blood in those disorienting days was driven by more than a wish to help the immediate victims of terrorism. The excessive nature of the donations—the queuing through the night, the reported reluctance to withdraw when no more storage space could be found, the continued high rates of donation after it was evident that there was far more blood available than could be used to treat the victims—this excess points to something more. It points, we argue, to the complex imbrication of giving blood with ideas and feelings about nation, citizenship and community, and the place of the body and its capacities within this constellation of concepts.

The technology of mass blood donation and transfusion has its origins in war and national defense. Blood banking methods were first developed in Barcelona during the Spanish Civil War,[2] and perfected in the United States, the United Kingdom, and Northern Africa during the Second World War. Small blood collection networks were set up in London and other British cities in the early days of the war. Physicians in the United States collected civilian blood to send to Britain, and the Free French created a facility in Algeria to assist their forces fighting in southern France and Corsica. In each location the citizenry came forward in large numbers to give blood for the troops as a fundamental contribution to the war effort. As Starr (1998) describes it, blood was both strategic matériel in the Allied war effort, a resource, and a substance associated with the values of democracy and anti-fascism. Giving blood was a way for civilians to participate in the sacrifice made by soldiers at the front, to defend the integrity of the nation by giving part of their bodies. Starr, commenting on the Free French approach to blood collection, observes, "To them it represented a philosophy of medical care, embodying all that was both modern and humane, especially in contrast to the values of the fascist enemy. Blood donation was benevolent, voluntary and welcomed from all, French and Arab alike. Blood thus became more than a pharmaceutical; it symbolized a new social contract" (Starr 1998, 154).

Giving blood to the troops was a way to express solidarity and improve morale in the anxious conditions of world war. As Rabinow comments, the relationship between blood donation, distribution, and the war effort gave a particular cast to the systems of civilian blood banking set up after the war, particularly in the United Kingdom and France: "After the war, transfusion carried with it the mark of solidarity, of a voluntary and benevolent gesture, of a collective effort of the entire nation" (Rabinow 1999, 84).

Thus blood donation, even in the United States, where postwar blood banking and donation practices diverged markedly from the nationalized, welfarist models favored in the United Kingdom and France, is historically associated with the bonds and obligations of citizenship and the defense of the nation,[3] an idea which in turn emerges from nineteenth-century ideas equating blood with race and race with national citizenship (Foucault 1980). In a sense, the anxious queues outside blood facilities in New York in the days after the World Trade Center attacks were formed by the first volunteers in a new war effort by the United States, albeit a war profoundly different from the Second World War.[4] This was war not with the standing army of another nation-state but with a globally organized, deterritorialized, and decentralized network of terrorist cells, who in attacking the World Trade Center and the Pentagon had managed to do what no national standing army had ever done—strike the mainland sovereign territory of the United States. The excessive desire to give blood was perhaps driven by a sense that the body politic was itself wounded in the attacks. Giving blood might help to heal the great visible trauma to lower Manhattan, the smoking ruins broadcast on national and international television for months hence.

The huge national mobilization of blood donors also suggests the continued currency of civic values often said to be in decline—values of altruism, citizenship, and identification with the fate of the nation over and above more segmented ethnic and religious identity. It suggests the continued currency of what Benedict Anderson famously called the imagined community of the nation-state, "Imagined because the members of even the smallest nation will never know most of their fellow members . . . yet in the minds of each lives the image of their communion. . . . it is imagined as community because, regardless of the actual inequality and exploitation that may prevail in each, the nation is always conceived as a deep, horizontal comradeship" (Anderson 1991, 6–7). For Anderson, citizens participate in fundamental acts of national imagined community when they read the national newspapers, and fight in national wars. Both acts involve citizens in a national narrative, and require them to imagine relations of solidarity with others in the space of the nation, others whom they will never meet. Blood donation too would appear to be an exemplary act of imagined community in Anderson's terms, a gift of health to an unknown other with whom one has nothing in common other than the shared space of the nation.

Numerous social theorists, particularly theorists of globalization, have argued that the kind of national imagined community posited by Anderson has fragmented irrevocably as the sovereign power of nation-states has been overtaken by deterritorialized social and political networks that characterize a globalized social order. As Urry (2000) articulates this shift, the new mobilities of people, capital, technologies, images, and ideas that characterize globalization have loosened the identification of citizens with the nation-state and diversified the forms of belonging and obligation available to organize citizenship. He writes,

> Global networks and flows restructure social inequalities and transform many states into [mere] regulators of such flows. Corporations, brands, NGOs and multinational 'states' have emerged more powerful than nation-states. . . . Overall the hybrid character of many apparent societies in a post-colonial period results in a disjunctive, contested and inconsistent citizenship . . . There are many social organizations delivering different kinds of rights and duties to different kinds of citizens over very different geographical reaches. Citizenship is contested not just within a nation-state over the access of different social groups to rights such as personal property, a job or health care. There is a more fundamental contestation over what are the appropriate rights and duties of citizens living within, and moving around, the contemporary world; over what entities should provide citizenship, and over what entities should adjudicate between the different complexes of rights and duties over very different temporal and spatial scales. (Urry 2000, 163)

According to this kind of analysis, the sense of belonging within a nationally bounded imaginary community that Anderson attributes to the modern citizen has not been effaced, but only complicated and attenuated by other emerging forms of obligation and identification. The intense national identifications evident in the World Trade Center blood donations are not artifacts of a bygone era of the nation-state but coexist with these other kinds of identification in an uneasy tension, available for mobilization under particular circumstances. The specificity of the September 11 donations, the immediate responsiveness of the donors to the plight of *these* citizens and to new conditions of warfare, coupled with poor national rates of regular blood donation, is evidence of these kinds of tensions.[5] The blood supply itself has been subject to complex international pressures over the last twenty years, which have disturbed any simple equation between the borders of the nation-state and the origins of transfusion blood. This is particularly true of the blood supply in the United States, which depends upon a more decentralized and privatized system than exists in the United Kingdom and most West European countries. Moreover, as we shall examine in detail, the contamination of the blood supply with human immunodeficiency virus (HIV) and hepatitis C virus (HCV) during the 1980s, due in part to the globalization of blood sources, has had a major impact on what blood means. The blood bank has been transformed from a source of communalized health to one of communalized risk, with parts of the population (sex workers, gay men, drug users) feared by other parts of the population as a source of contaminated blood (Waldby et al. 2004). Nevertheless, blood donation evidently retains powers of national mobilization and the power to express public health as a collective enterprise, shared among fellow citizens under particular circumstances.

Tissue Transfer and Social Order The World Trade Center attacks reminded many Americans that blood is a substance capable of being transferred between people, but in fact the disaster forced the mobilization of all sorts of body parts and biomedical technologies for their transfer and analysis. So for example, in the days following the attacks skin banks sent several square meters of allograft skin to New York City for burn victims. For many months afterward, volunteers and crisis workers searched the ruins for often tiny fragments of human remains, some identifiable remnant of the victims who were being mourned. Forensics experts used computers to analyze the fragments' DNA, sometimes even creating new software programs able to identify individuals on the basis of short single-nucleotide polymorphisms (SNPS).[6]

The medical response to the World Trade Center attacks, in other words, was closely linked to the affective significance of human tissues, their ability to represent complex ideas and feelings about human identity and community. The response also drew on extensive technical systems for the donation, circulation, analysis, and transplantation of human tissues available now, in the first years of the twenty-first century. While blood transfusion has been routinely practiced for one hundred years, other kinds of tissue transplantation are much more recent (we use "tissue" throughout this book in a generic sense, to include blood, organs, and any other kind of living matter taken from the body). Solid organ transplantation has been practiced since the late 1950s and commonplace since the late 1970s, as the refinement of tissue typing, surgical techniques, and immunological suppression has allowed organ donors to be matched with compatible recipients (Fox and Swazey 1992). Skin, bone, heart valves, and corneas can now be banked and used in surgery (Hurley 1995). Reproductive tissue—sperm, ova, and embryos—can be donated and transplanted. Umbilical cord blood is increasingly harvested during birth procedures, stored, and used as an alternative to bone marrow in transplants. The recent development of techniques for propagating human stem cell lines derived from embryos means that embryonic tissues may become the source for a completely new range of transplantable tissues sometime in the future (Waldby 2002a). Many other kinds of tissues—cancerous material, surgical waste, saliva samples—are banked for medical research or commercial pharmaceutical production. Currently several countries, including Iceland, Singapore, Estonia, Sweden, the United Kingdom, and Canada, are setting up genetic databases that will contain DNA data about a substantial share of their populations (Kaye 2004a).

This proliferation of tissue fragments, and of medical and social technologies for their sourcing, storage, and distribution, has profound implications for health and embodiment, for civil identity and social order, and for delineating relations between the global and the local. Each new technology involves a reorganization of the boundaries and elements of the human body, the development of new kinds of "separable, exchangeable and reincorporable body parts" (Rabinow 1999, 95). What does it mean when the human body can be disaggregated into fragments that are derived from a particular person but are, strictly speaking, no longer constitutive of human identity (Rabinow 1999)? What is the legal status of such fragments? Are they a kind of property in the body? Does the person from whom they originate have defensible claims over them once they enter into social circulation? Are they experienced as fragments of the donor's self after donation, or as detachable objects (Waldby et al. 2004)? Do donors and recipients feel that some enduring relationship is created between them in the act of tissue transfer (Waldby 2002b)? How is the status of the individual (strictly speaking the in-*dividual*, he who cannot be subdivided) altered to accommodate these possibilities for fragmentation?

At the level of social relations, how might the exchange of such fragments between persons, their donation or sale, their receipt and reincorporation, constitute relationships between them? The sharing of human tissues can be a powerful expression of communal solidarity and civil empathy, as we have already seen. However, the redistribution of human tissues can also produce injustice and exploitation, because one person makes a bodily sacrifice in favor of another's health and life. Often the transfer of tissues from one person to another follows the trajectories of power and wealth, as the poor sell their body parts to those with more wealth. The increased global mobility of people and money has seen the growth, alongside carefully regulated national systems for organ donation, of transnational black markets in human organs, sold by the urban and rural poor of the developing nations to aging, wealthy buyers in the industrialized world (Scheper-Hughes 2000). Thus the biotechnical capacity to transfer tissues immediately raises questions of just distribution. What social technologies and forms of governance are the most appropriate for this task? What complexities are introduced into all of these questions by the increasing globalization and liberalizing of the market in human tissue? Biotechnology and pharmaceutical companies are international brokers of many kinds of human tissue—stem cells, genetic material, blood products—and play an increasingly powerful role in shaping national health policy. How do these developments interact with older models of a national commitment to public health, and the free donation of tissues to fellow citizens?

The medical capacity to fragment the body and the techno-social systems that manage and distribute these fragments, in other words, raise fundamental issues about ontology, power, economy, and community, some of which we hope to address in this book. We propose to tackle these issues through a critical appraisal of the dichotomy that has organized bioethical and sociological evaluations of these issues for the last thirty years—the dichotomy of gift and commodity. Makers of health policy in the United Kingdom have favored, for the most part, a gift model for managing human tissues—that is, a model in which donation is voluntary, without financial compensation, and distribution is based on medical need rather than ability to pay. In the United States gift and commodity systems for some human tissues exist side by side—for example in reproductive material, which can be both donated and sold—while others, for example whole organs, are circulated strictly as gifts.

Advocates for the greater commodification of therapeutic tissues generally base their arguments on the efficacy of the market as a way to increase the number of organ or blood donors through financial reward. Their arguments are pragmatic and utilitarian, advocating payment for kidneys, for example, as a way to increase supply.[7] Advocates of gift systems, however, claim a much wider ambit of social benefits. As Rabinow (1999) reports, French bioethical deliberations and legal constraints prohibit the selling of human tissues, on the grounds that the commercialization of tissues is incompatible with human dignity, a bioethical position shared by institutions in the United Kingdom and those of many other countries to a greater or lesser extent. As we have already seen, the gift of blood is historically associated with the constitution of a community-minded citizenry and a resilient nation, a claim examined in detail below and throughout the book. Correlatively, the advocates of gift systems associate the selling of human tissues with exploitation and dehumanization, the reduction of human status to the status of a thing (Andrews and Nelkin 2001; Scheper-Hughes 2000; Kimbrell 1993). Scheper-Hughes, for example, likens the commodification of organs to "a new form of late modern cannibalism": "Commercialized transplant medicine has allowed global society to be divided into two decidedly unequal populations—organ givers and organ receivers. The former are an invisible and discredited collection of anonymous suppliers of spare parts; the latter are cherished patients, treated as moral subjects and suffering individuals. Their names and their biographies and medical histories are known, and their proprietary rights over the bodies and body parts of the poor, living and dead, are virtually unquestioned" (Scheper-Hughes 2002a, 4).

Gift systems and commodity systems for managing human tissues are often cast in this way, as mutually exclusive and morally incompatible social forms. In this book we hope to complicate and disorganize the gift-commodity dichotomy, because we consider it an inadequate way to conceptualize the political economy of tissues in the modern world of globalized biotechnology. To do this we will first consider the most eloquent theorization of the relationships between gift and commodity systems of tissue exchange and their implications for citizenship, identity, community, the body, and the body politic: Richard Titmuss's celebrated study *The Gift Relationship: From Human Blood to Social Policy*, first published in 1970. Titmuss, a great scholar and defender of the postwar welfare state, sets out a compelling set of arguments for retaining a gift model for blood donation and transfusion. We will first consider his arguments in some detail. We will then consider the impact of subsequent developments in biotechnology, commerce, globalization, and social theory on the specific content of his arguments.

Titmuss: The Political Economy of Tissues Titmuss's work is inescapable because he recognized that the material forms of tissue circulation have complex implications for the form of the polity. *The Gift Relationship*, written in the late 1960s, is a primarily comparative study of the systems of blood donation and distribution that grew up after the Second World War in the United Kingdom and the United States. These two systems served Titmuss as exemplars of the virtues of the gift over the commodity form, and of public over market models of service provision. At the time when Titmuss was writing, the British blood system retained much of the character of the wartime service. As part of the postwar creation of a comprehensive National Health Service (NHS), a National Blood Service (NBS) was set up under the jurisdiction of the Ministry of Health. Blood was treated along the lines of the nationalized health system and the postwar welfare state reforms, as a public resource to be distributed according to social principles of capacity to give and medical need. Donors gave without remuneration, as they had during the war, and a system of regional transfusion centers ensured that each hospital in a region was supplied according to need. Patients did not pay for blood received, nor were they obliged to give blood in return. The system was entirely voluntary (Starr 1998). Despite the rapid increase in demand for blood attendant on new forms of surgery, this voluntary system provided an adequate supply of blood during the years leading up to Titmuss's study. Between 1951 and 1965 almost every regional center increased the size of its donor pool (Titmuss 1997).

In the United States, in the absence of any national policy on blood management, a much more complex and internally conflicted set of arrangements grew up to supply hospitals with blood. During the war the Red Cross had been the primary coordinator of the blood mobilization effort, though small local and community blood banks had also opened to meet the demand. After the war these two forms of organization continued to coexist, despite attempts by the Red Cross to establish itself as the sole national blood supplier. The Red Cross managed a system that more closely resembled the British one, with predominantly free voluntary donation and transfusion, while the community blood banks often used a credit system according to which recipients of transfusion owed the bank a donation, from either themselves or a friend or relative. Both systems would on occasion use paid donors to supplement voluntary ones. They did so reluctantly, on the grounds that people who sold blood were more likely than voluntary donors to present a risk of hepatitis or syphilis. Unable to cooperate, the two systems divided the United States into an erratic patchwork of territories, and patients might find themselves in either a voluntary or a credit system according to where they fell ill. Excesses and deficiencies in regional blood supply could not be remedied, because neither service would share information with the other, leading to much wastage (Starr 1998).

In addition to this confusion, a parallel system of for-profit blood banks grew up alongside the voluntary sector during the 1950s, exploiting the gaps and problems in supply and demand arising from regional and organizational conflicts. In the absence of a licensing system, nonmedical entrepreneurs could set up a bank with a minimal degree of medical supervision, buy blood (often from the poor and derelict), and sell it to hospitals. During the early 1960s the worst implications of this unregulated market for blood played out in a spectacular legal battle in the Federal Trade Commission (FTC), a legal battle that strongly influenced Titmuss's thinking about the pivotal status of blood in forming social relations. In an action initiated by the for-profit blood banks in Kansas City, the FTC investigated the charge that the city's community blood banks were engaged in an illegal trade boycott of the commercial sector by refusing to purchase blood from it. At the heart of the case was this question: Was blood a commodity, or did it have some other kind of status? At its initial hearing the FTC accepted the argument that because citrate anticoagulant was added to blood to increase its shelf life, blood was not simply a living human substance but a commodity, "something that could be bought, sold and processed like any other drug. As such it would fall subject to the normal trade laws, forbidding economic boycotts and restraint of trade" (Starr 1998, 228). The implications of this for the community suppliers were both that they would be obliged to purchase blood that they considered a public health risk and that any recipient of tainted blood (still a very real possibility under the strictest testing and hygiene regimes available at the time) could sue the suppliers for violating implied warranty. The community sector appealed, and in 1969 the FTC decided that the case, since it involved nonprofit groups, did not come under its jurisdiction. The potential to treat blood as a commodity was not restricted by the ruling, and in the late 1960s another form of for-profit blood business developed. Pharmaceutical companies set up plasma collection businesses using a technique called plasmapheresis, which enabled the collection of large amounts of plasma from paid donors, to be used in the production of blood products. Again the donor populations were predominantly the indigent and homeless, and the pooling of the collected plasma in large vats presented a serious risk of contamination.

Mindful of these developments, Titmuss set out to defend the British voluntary system of blood donation against the dangers that he saw in the quasi-commercial system of the United States. Titmuss believed that the greatest threat to the gift system was not the pragmatic example of the blood system in the United States per se but the early stirrings of neoliberal market rationalism, articulated by economists like Friedrich von Hayek and Milton Friedman. His particular target was the policies favored by the influential Institute of Economic Affairs (IEA), a neoconservative think tank,[8] which advocated introducing market forces and analysis into British health care (Fontaine 2002). Titmuss regarded its arguments as a serious challenge to the National Health Service and its philosophy of national community and distributive justice. More broadly, he saw market rationalism as imperiling the whole ethos of welfare and public provision which characterized postwar Britain and which he considered essential to social cohesion. As

Philippe Fontaine comments in his detailed analysis of the historical context of Titmuss's work, "Encouraged by Labour's return to power in 1964 . . . [Titmuss] reconsidered the orientation of social policy in connection with externalities—that is, benefits and costs that are external to the market and for which people neither pay nor are compensated. In Titmuss's view, 'socialist' social policies stimulated ethical behavior, which generates positive externalities and averts negative externalities, whereas 'private' social policies, as envisaged by the IEA, favored commercialism, which neglects positive externalities and underestimates negative externalities. . . . Titmuss could sense that economic considerations were gaining ground in official Labour circles, a trend that would lead to gradual departures from the principle of free social services in the second half of the 1960s" (Fontaine 2002, 403).

Titmuss's intention in writing *The Gift Relationship* was to demonstrate how the problems evident in the American system typified the danger of exposing essential human services like blood donation to market forces (Oakley and Ashton 1997). The book contains a thorough investigation of the size and composition of donor pools, contamination risks, and blood wastage in each system. It found that the voluntary, national system in the United Kingdom provided a donor pool drawn from all social classes, better security against infectious contamination, and little wastage of blood supplies. The system in the United States, on the other hand, drew a high proportion of its ever-dwindling donor pool from ill and indigent donors, and the fragmentation of the system produced high degrees of waste and expense. More importantly for us, Titmuss used these findings to formulate a complex and rigorous argument about the values of the social as opposed to the economic sphere of life, and the moral and civil effects of gift systems of tissue circulation, which he opposed to commodity systems. In doing so he set out a framework for thinking about tissue donation and banking that is still highly influential in bioethical and health policy arenas throughout the world.

Titmuss locates the donation and distribution of blood within a broader set of questions regarding the nature of the social contract and the power of the welfare state to produce egalitarian and communitarian relations between citizens. At the start of *The Gift Relationship*, he notes:

[This] study originates . . . from a series of value questions formulated within the context of attempts to distinguish the "social" from the "economic" in public policies and in those institutions and services with declared welfare goals. Could, however, such distinctions be drawn and the territory of social policy at least broadly defined without raising issues about the morality of society and of man's regard or disregard for the needs of others? Why should men not contract out of the social and act to their own immediate advantage? Why give to strangers?—a question that provokes an even more fundamental moral issue: who is my stranger in the relatively affluent, acquisitive and divisive societies of the twentieth century? What are the connections then, if obligations are extended, between the reciprocals of giving and receiving and modern welfare systems? (Titmuss 1997, 57–58)

For Titmuss the management of blood is a critical nodal point in the network of civil obligations created by a democratic welfare state. If blood, as an intimate part of the embodied self, is not sequestered from market forces, then all kinds of social services—education, social security, child foster care, social work—would also inevitably be laid open to the market, because the sharing rather than selling of blood represents *the* fundamental assertion of collective values. "To give or not to give, to lend, repay or even buy and sell blood leads us . . . into the fundamentals of social and economic life" (Titmuss 1997, 124). Blood must be given and not sold, Titmuss writes, because the circulation of gifts is crucial to forming collective social relations and mutuality among citizens. He develops this argument by drawing on Marcel Mauss's celebrated anthropological study of gift relations in Melanesian, Polynesian, and Canadian Indian societies, *The Gift: The Form and Reason for Exchange in Archaic Societies*. Mauss identified the giving and receiving of gifts as the primary basis for social solidarity in these societies. Gifts are important, Mauss argues, because they create relations of indebtedness and obligation between parties. Gifts are not so much things as relationships between persons. A gift exercises a certain hold over its recipient, insofar as the recipient is bound to the giver by the obligation to reciprocate. In this sense the gift is not a simple transfer of ownership from one party to another, but instead invokes the person of the giver, even after it has been given. Mauss writes, "What imposes obligation in the [gift] received and exchanged, is the fact that the thing received is not inactive. Even when it has been abandoned by the giver, it still possesses something of him. Through it the giver has a hold over the beneficiary . . . to make a gift of something to someone is to make a present of some part of oneself . . . [and] to accept something from someone is to accept some part of his spiritual essence, his soul" (Mauss 1990, 11–12).

Frow (1997), in his careful reading of Mauss, notes that in this traditional system of obligatory giving, receiving, and reciprocation, gifts act more like loans. They both create and mediate relationships between persons, and continue to refer to their original owner, irrespective of circulation. They create above all a demand and obligation for reciprocation, and so the circulation of gifts creates a web of indebtedness and exerts a continued pressure for reciprocity. "The gift continues to form a part of the giver even when alienated to another . . . this link is a kind of property right which persists as an obligation to return the gift, even when the gift passes through a number of hands. We are concerned here with a transaction that perhaps bears rather more resemblance to a loan than to an absolute gift or the alienation of a property right" (Frow 1997, 110).

It is this power of gifts to constitute positive social relations that Titmuss draws upon to argue for the necessity of voluntary and gratuitous blood donation. Titmuss notes that in traditional societies, strict forms of obligation and compulsion characterize gift relations. As displays of wealth, they are crucial for creating chiefly hierarchies and personal power. Gift giving in this context is not disinterested and altruistic, but rather caught up in a system of calculation and strategy. Titmuss argues, however, that the gift of blood in the modern welfare state is a different category of practice. It is free of power relationships because it is impersonal, transmitted from one stranger to another, and so lacks the element of personal aggrandizement and indebtedness. It is voluntary, not compulsory, and the recipient is under no personal pressure to reciprocate. It is given not because the giver expects a return, but as an act of voluntary altruism and social duty. Blood is both an intimate part of a person and a circulable substance that can be given to another under conditions of mutual anonymity. Hence giving and receiving blood create the conditions for imagined community (Anderson 1991) among fellow citizens, a sense of impersonal mutuality and inclusion, in place of the personal relations of power and indebtedness described by Mauss. Rather than constitute complex forms of social hierarchy, the gift of blood, according to Titmuss's model, helps to constitute a sense of social responsibility and trust among strangers, and gratitude not toward particular persons but to the social body as a whole. As social policy, free blood donation forms an integrative system, in which "[p]rocesses, transactions and institutions . . . promote an individual's sense of identity, participation and community and allow him more freedom of choice for the expression of altruism and . . . discourage a sense of individual alienation" (Titmuss 1997, 20). Furthermore, this system promotes good public health. In a nonremunerative system, donors have no profit incentive to lie about their health. They are much more likely than paid donors, for example, to truthfully answer questions about past episodes of hepatitis or syphilis. A gift system also promotes equitable redistribution, transferring precious biological matériel from the healthy to the ill, the strong to the weak, along the same lines of economy as those associated with the welfare state. In this way the blood bank becomes a site for constituting both collective health and the best values of citizenship, where the bodies of citizens are materially indebted to each other and to the redistributive state.

So for Titmuss, organizing blood along the lines of a gift system was a way to engender socially constructive and redistributive embodied relations between citizens. A gift economy for blood, he believed, would promote the optimum form of circulation to maintain the body politic of the welfare state, by creating a particular kind of civil intercorporeality, one in which the explicit relations of indebtedness between bodies would provoke a continued round of donation, a continuing replenishment of both the population's vitality and its generosity. Titmuss explicitly contrasts this communitarian economy with the social fragmentation that he believed was produced by the marketization of blood, its exposure to pricing mechanisms. Markets, he claimed, organize oppositional relationships between buyers and sellers, and resolve this opposition through the striking of price and the completion of a transaction. Selling blood creates instrumental, nonbinding commodity relations between producers and consumers, whose relationship is strictly temporary, lasting as long as the transaction. If blood is subject to market relations then the identity between the person and his or her blood is severed, so that it circulates as a commodity and is incorporated as an object of possession and consumption, without the creation of any tie between vendor and purchaser. On the contrary, any relationship can be readily disentangled, as the blood itself is decontextualized from its point of production. As Frow puts it, "a market system . . . puts in place some very specific negative freedoms: freedom from obligation to or for unnamed strangers, and freedom from a sense of inclusion in the social" (Frow 1997, 105). It allows individuals to contract out of the social, to act in purely instrumental ways that further their own self-interest, including the selling of their blood to the highest bidder. The commodification of such an intimate part of the person was for Titmuss a synecdoche for the reduction of all forms of relationship to the contractual mechanisms of capitalism, and the destruction of any domain of social life outside of market relations. It is, he implies, on a continuum with slavery, the commodification not of the body as a whole but of body parts: "Short of examining . . . the institution of slavery—of men and women as market commodities—blood as a living tissue may now constitute in Western societies one of the ultimate tests of where the 'social' begins and the 'economic' ends. If blood is considered . . . as a trading commodity, then ultimately human hearts, kidneys, eyes and other organs of the body may also come to be treated as commodities to be bought and sold in the marketplace" (Titmuss 1997, 219).

The commodification of blood is also detrimental to public and individual health and to the proper delivery of health services. Drawing on the Kansas City case described above, Titmuss argues that establishing a market in blood would bring all blood-related medicine under the purview of commercial law: "A private market in blood . . . or other sectors of medical care will, in the end, require to be supported and controlled by the same laws of restraint and warranty as those that obtain in the buying and selling of consumption goods" (Titmuss 1997, 230). The blood sector would become the domain of civil litigation and adversarial relations between doctors and patients. Marketizing blood also distributes blood from the poor, who need to sell their blood, to the rich, who can afford to pay for it. It draws on a necessarily less healthy population, and if blood has a price, this gives the donor an incentive to lie about his or her health. Hence Titmuss regards paid donors as presenting a greater risk of introducing infection, particularly serum hepatitis, into the blood supply: "The paid seller of blood is confronted . . . with a personal conflict of interests. To tell the truth about himself, his way of life and his relationships may limit his freedom to sell his blood in the market. Because he desires money and is not seeking in this particular act to affirm a sense of belonging, he thinks primarily of his own freedom; he separates his freedom from other people's freedoms" (Titmuss 1997, 308). Titmuss concludes his study with a round condemnation of blood markets:

> From our study of the private market in blood in the United States, we have concluded that the commercialization of blood and donor relationships represses the expression of altruism, erodes the sense of community, lowers scientific standards, limits both personal and professional freedoms, sanctions the making of profits in clinics and laboratories, legalizes hostility between doctor and patient, subjects critical areas of medicine to the laws of the marketplace, places immense social costs on those least able to bear them—the poor, the sick and the inept—increases the dangers of unethical behavior in various sectors of medical science and practice, and results in situations in which proportionally more and more blood is supplied by the poor, the unskilled and the unemployed, Negroes and other low income groups and categories of exploited populations of high blood yielders. Redistribution of blood and blood products from the poor to the rich appears to be one of the dominant effects of the American blood-banking systems. (Titmuss 1997, 314)

The Social, the Economic, and the Body Titmuss's study conceptualizes tissue distribution systems as specific political economies with intrinsic forms of value, exchange, and circulation, and the power to constitute sociality. It retains the fundamental insight of Marx's work on capital and the commodity form: that gifts and commodities "are not objects at all, but transactions and social relations. . . . As an order of social relations the gift economy [and the commodity economy are] bound up with the forms of the person as they are diversely constituted and as it constitutes them" (Frow 1997, 124). Titmuss's primary concern is to formulate social policies that protect a putative realm of social values and "social man" against the predations of the market and "economic man." His passionate defense of the gift of blood is an attempt to insert the human body as a wedge between encroaching marketization and a domain of nonmarket sociality, where, he believes, social relations can be purely qualitative and free of calculation. In arguing that blood must be anonymously given and accepted, not bought and sold, Titmuss attempts to consolidate the principle that the human body, and the forms of sociality built upon its capacities, exist beyond relations of commerce, and that the value of the body is intrinsic and unquantifiable. Only an unqualified and unquantified civil generosity, the direct sharing of bodily substance, would adequately maintain the material relations of the welfare state and guard against the dehumanizing, fragmenting action of corporeal markets.

Here Titmuss draws on a discourse regarding the dignity of the human body that developed in an international context after the disclosure of the atrocities committed during the Second World War. A number of documents related to the establishment of international human rights legislation, including the Universal Declaration of Human Rights (1948) and the International Covenant on Civil and Political Rights (1966), employ the term "dignity" as defining the status of humans (Schachter 1983). As Rabinow (1999) notes, this contemporary understanding of dignity draws heavily on the Kantian opposition between dignity and price, or absolute and relative value: "In the kingdom of ends everything has either a price or a dignity. Whatever has a price can be replaced by something else as its equivalent; on the other hand, whatever is above all price, and therefore admits of no equivalent, has a dignity" (Kant 1981, 40). Working from this opposition between price and dignity, many twentieth-century politicians and bioethicists argued that the human body itself is the locus of absolute dignity, and that dignity involves the preservation and protection of integrity. Dignity is destroyed if any part of the body is assigned a market value and rendered alienable.

Using this international moral conceptualization, Titmuss could position the absolute value of the body and its products as the most effective and worthy bulwark against the incipient commercial forces that he felt threatened the postwar welfare state. As we have seen, Titmuss wrote *The Gift Relationship* as a direct rejoinder to the early articulations of neoliberal economics, and published it just at the point when the postwar social consensus in favor of a Keynesian, welfarist nation-state, understood as a protection against both communism and the economic instability of the Great Depression, began to fracture. A few years after the publication in 1970 of *The Gift Relationship*, the international economic order began to shift irrevocably, a shift highlighted by the oil crisis, the end of the Bretton Woods agreement and the gold standard, and the decline of industrial production in favor of "informational" and service production as the economic base for the advanced industrial economies. The postwar welfare state was gradually undermined in ways that Titmuss had partially foreseen. By the early 1980s neoliberal administrations in the United States and Britain were actively devolving state provision of pensions and health services to the private sector, privatizing previously "essential" public infrastructure like telecommunications and energy, shrinking the tax base and shifting the economic base from nationally organized industry to transnational finance capital.

At the same time, blood plasma processing became an international business operated by increasingly powerful pharmaceutical multinationals. These companies used paid donors, often the poor in underdeveloped countries, to meet the blood requirements of the industrialized nations. We investigate this development at length in chapter 1. Here we can see the beginnings of the biocommercial activity that was to become such an important part of international commerce in the 1980s and 1990s, one of the primary drivers of the new knowledge economies. Titmuss's text linked these two phenomena, the commodification of human tissues and the neoliberalization of economies. In his argument, the commodification of human tissues leads irrevocably to the decline of the welfare state. Enshrining the noncommodifiable status of the body was, he thought, the best hedge against such a decline.

Yet even as the postwar welfare state was showing signs of collapse, *The Gift Relationship* proved to be a very influential book. It prompted the Nixon administration to begin reforms of the blood donation system and to decrease, although not eliminate, paid donors for whole blood. Margaret Thatcher's failure to marketize the blood donation system in Britain has been linked to the success and popularity of the book's arguments among doctors and health administrators (Oakley and Ashton 1997). Titmuss's ideas inform present policies in the United Kingdom regarding other kinds of human tissue. As in western Europe and the industrialized Commonwealth countries (Canada, Australia, New Zealand), donors may not sell their tissues:[9] generally speaking, human tissues must be given (Medical Research Council 2001; Council of Europe 1997). In the United States in the mid-1980s, Titmuss's book was cited approvingly in congressional hearings that eventually resulted in the prohibition of whole organ sales.

Tissue Economies in the Information Age   Titmuss's study of blood donation provides us with a dynamic, open-ended set of concepts about the social constitution of tissue economies, one that can be productively linked to contemporary theoretical and political concerns. It speaks very directly to the social, philosophical, and feminist literatures on embodiment, for it understands tissue donation as a way to constitute relationships between embodied citizens, to develop public trust and social equity through systems for the exchange of bodily substance. Tissue donation also expresses the way the populace is related to the nation-state: people donate because they identify themselves as included in the common fate of the nation. Titmuss's study also provides ways to analyze relationships between different systems for sourcing, distributing, and incorporating human tissues and to understand the consequences of each for public and individual health, social justice, and subjectivity. In positing and elaborating these relationships, Titmuss's work is invaluable for any attempt to understand what is at stake in contemporary tissue economies.

However, we would argue that Titmuss's study also has some significant limitations and blind spots, particularly evident when his argument is applied to more recent developments in tissue exchange. In particular, his reliance on what he considered the inherent moral and distributive qualities of gift systems as a solution to all potential problems is no longer an adequate response. Recent biotechnical, economic, and critical developments render the specific content of

Titmuss's approach problematic in several ways. First, Titmuss represented the gift of blood as a relatively simple *transfer* of a stable substance—*whole* blood—from one person to another, a representation that enhanced his model of anonymous generosity and exchange between equal strangers. However, very soon after the publication of *The Gift Relationship*, the technologies of blood transfusion changed. Since the mid-1970s a donated unit has generally been fractioned into a number of components—plasma, red cells, white cells, and platelets—and rarely transfused as whole blood. Hence one donor's blood may go to several recipients in some form, and a single recipient may receive blood products from more than one donor. This form of circulation somewhat complicates Titmuss's emphasis on blood as a one-to-one transaction between subjects, and indicates a disjuncture between the technical systems for the circulation of blood and the social economies of citizenship. Many contemporary tissue economies are still more complex and fractured than those of blood donation, further emphasizing this disjuncture. The engineering of tissues after donation means that any donated tissue may be put to multiple uses and adopt multiple trajectories (Waldby 2002a). With the exception of some organs, donated tissues are not simply transferred intact from one person to another, but rather diverted through laboratory processes where they may be fractionated, cloned, immortalized, and multiplied in various ways. Tissue sourced from one person may be distributed in altered forms along complex pathways to multiple recipients at different times and at different locations throughout the world. So, for example, a single donated embryo may form the starting point for several immortalized cell lines that can be copied, divided, sent to laboratories and clinics around the world, and eventually used to treat an open-ended number of patients. Tissue donation is thus transformed from an act of direct civic responsibility between fellow citizens into a complex network of donor-recipient relations heavily mediated by biotechnical processes and an institutional complex of tissue banks, pharmaceutical and research companies, and clinics. The implications of these networks for the social relations of tissue exchange will form one of the overarching themes of this book.

Second, the increasingly global nature of tissue exchanges renders problematic any attempts to isolate national medical systems from international systems of exchange. While Titmuss's study was primarily concerned with whole blood, a substance whose relatively short shelf life means that it tends to be collected and distributed within national boundaries, blood products like plasma and Factor VIII, a treatment for hemophilia, are sourced globally and processed and sold by transnational pharmaceutical companies. Sperm banks like the Scandinavian Cryobank set up international branches to market "Nordic" semen to women in the United States and elsewhere.[10] The embryonic stem cell lines described above are another instance of tissue fragments that circulate across borders and between laboratories, tissue banks, and bodies in complex systems that exceed the regulations of any nation-state, and can rapidly disseminate both vital life-giving matter and contamination risks throughout the world. Hence the movement of tissues from one body to another is likely to take place beyond the relationships characterized by national citizenship and the body of law and governance that regulates national space. The difficulties of regulating transnational tissue exchange are manifested most urgently in the growth of global black markets for kidneys or corneas from live donors, who sell their body's long-term capacities for cash (Scheper-Hughes 2002a). How can we characterize the diversity of transnational interactions created by this proliferation and complication of global tissue economies?

Third, Titmuss's work, like most subsequent bioethical work, enshrines the principle that the human body exists beyond relations of commerce, and that its value is intrinsic and unquantifiable. In this it reflects both the Kantian discourse of dignity, discussed above, and the English common-law principle that persons do not have a property right in their bodies, and hence cannot sell themselves or purchase another. Since the publication of Titmuss's study, this laudable principle has become vexed in the area of tissue donation by the rapidly increasing commercial value of the tissue fragment *after it has been donated*. While donors are largely excluded in U.S. and British law from selling their tissues (with the exception of reproductive tissues and plasma in the United States), their donated tissue may be either sold by the receiving party (hospitals routinely sell tissues to pharmaceutical or cosmetics companies, for example) or transformed into cell lines or gene sequences and patented. The extension of intellectual property rights to living entities has had a decisive effect on the biopolitics of human tissues. In the case of *Diamond v. Chakrabarty* (1980), discussed in chapter 3, the U.S. Supreme Court allowed the granting of a patent for a genetically engineered bacterium, on the grounds that the critical distinction in intellectual property rights was not between living and nonliving entities but between natural and fabricated entities. Since then intellectual property rights have been established in multicellular entities like knockout mice, in immortalized cell lines based on adult human tissue, in embryonic stem cell lines, and in genetic sequences. This constitution of biological entities as the repositories of intellectual property has transformed biomedical research into a lucrative area of investment for the increasingly mobile forms of finance and venture capital that have dominated the global economy since the 1970s (Arrighi 1994). These novel forms of living matter thus become the material base for highly inventive kinds of biocommerce, and companies like Geron, Advanced Cell Technologies, PPL Therapeutics, and many others use their patent licensing rights to attract venture capital. At the same time, as we explore in detail in chapters 2 and 3, donors themselves are legally excluded from any stake in this profitability. This legal distribution of property rights raises serious questions of social equity unforeseen by Titmuss's endorsement of gratuitous donation as intrinsically ethical. Effectively his strategy to make the human body a bulwark against the commodification of social life, a strategy now institutionalized in bioethical procedure, has simply rendered the body an open source of free biological material for commercial use.

Fourth, recent anthropological, sociological, and legal work on structures of exchange has begun a major reevaluation of the seemingly mutually exclusive relationship between gifts and commodities assumed by Titmuss. Frow (1997), in his extended essay on gift and commodity forms, undertakes a thorough critique of the Marxist analysis, assumed by Titmuss, that the commodity form and the functions of the market have an a priori atomizing effect on human relations, while gift systems are inherently more ethical. After reviewing anthropological studies of both traditional and contemporary gift economies, and noting the extent to which gifts work to constitute power relations and to further various strategies of prestige and domination, he argues, "There is no single form of 'the gift,' and no pure type of either the gift economy or the commodity economy. . . . on the one hand gift and commodity economies are always intertwined in various hybrid configurations and present a range of alternative possibilities for the use of objects; on the other, gift and commodity are not mutually exclusive modes of transaction, since they tend to have in common certain forms of calculation, strategy, and motivation. The gift therefore cannot and should not be conceived as an ethical category: it embodies no general principle of creativity, of generosity, of gratuitous reciprocality, or of sacrifice or loss" (Frow 1997, 124).

Callon (1998) extends some of these points when he argues that in a complex contemporary economy, gift and commodity systems interpenetrate each other in increasingly complex ways, and cannot maintain mutually exclusive forms of social space or spheres of relationship. Markets do not form discrete spaces contained by the power of nonmarket regulatory institutions and social life, nor can gift relationships function free of market calculation or considerations of exchange value. As we shall see, this interpenetration of public and commercial agencies characterizes contemporary tissue economies and their products. Correlatively, the distinction made by Titmuss regarding the natures of "economic man" and "social man" is unsustainable, because it assumes "the existence of individual agents with perfectly stabilized competencies . . . endowed with a set of fixed interests and stable preferences" (Callon 1998, 8). Such fixed ontologies could not be maintained under the conditions of uncertainty, fluctuation, and demand for strategic calculation that characterize the social networks of modernity.

Moreover, according to work by Appadurai (1986) on the social life of things, an alleged discreteness between gift and commodity forms cannot secure discrete spheres of social and economic life, because the same object may change status from gift to commodity and back again, according to the network of relationships in which it circulates at any given time: "The commodity is not one kind of thing rather than another, but one phase in the life of some things" (Appadurai 1986, 17). Appadurai notes that societies place limitations and termination points on the commodification of certain sacred objects (relics, ritual items, etc.). A variety of human tissues falls into this category. Many people in the industrial democracies believe that embryos have a privileged relationship to the origins of human life, the opposite pole to the commodity (Kopytoff 1986; Waldby and Squier 2003). Other tissues—hair, urine, or saliva—have been historically treated as "abjects" that may be readily commodified precisely because they are waste, and do not signify the donor. As we shall see in chapter 2, the status of embryos is bitterly contested in many nations with active stem cell research programs, and embryos and the cell lines derived from them move in complex ways through gift and commodity regimes. Waste tissues have also changed status in dramatic ways under the aegis of genetic biotechnology, which can transform even the most modest biological material into both a marker for the self and a potentially lucrative source of genetic material or biological chemicals. We will examine some contestations and reversals of waste status in part II. Such rapid transformations of status, in and out of waste, gift, and commodity forms, typify the forms of circulating value assumed by human tissues today.

Finally, we point to the increasing importance of "information" as a mediating term between individuals and tissues used for research and therapies. The transformation of the economic foundation of the United States and most western European countries from industrial to informational has encouraged the extension of intellectual property categories (copyrights, patents, trademarks, and publicity rights) to an ever-increasing number of objects, and human tissues (and information about human tissues) are no exception. As a consequence, national courts and legislatures have become increasingly interested in understanding, and controlling, how informational flows—especially those between universities and corporations—operate in these countries. Models of public and national health still rely on the notion of individual donations of tissues, but these gifts are understood as components of vast informational systems that connect the public and corporate spheres both nationally and globally.

In what follows, we will examine some of the consequences of these transformations both in the socio-technical organization of tissue economies and in analytic frameworks for their understanding. It would be impossible today to account for all kinds of tissue economy in one book, so we have elected to explore case studies, described below, as indications of some broader trends.

This is a comparative study in two senses. First, we develop some general ideas about the concept of tissue economies, and the organization and transformations of tissue value, by comparing the social trajectories of different tissue types and their transformations over time. Second, like Titmuss we focus our study primarily on cases drawn from the United Kingdom and the United States. While we touch upon other national situations as we go, the regulatory complexities and national traditions in tissue management vary so much in their detail that it was imperative to settle on specific social locations. Titmuss began with the understanding that the United Kingdom and the United States had distinctly different approaches to valuating and managing human tissues, the first committed to gift economies and national health as a common public good, the second accommodating a mixed economy in which gifts and commodities, private and public health services, mingled and collided. We have retained his focus here, not because this distinction holds up in any clear way in practice, but because specific tissue economies in each location must navigate their way through these differing traditions and different cultural weightings placed on the gift and commodity forms. Because we investigate several tissue types, and because we are interested in the ways that ideas and practices of value mutate across different social and technical landscapes, our study is not rigorously and exhaustively comparative in an empirical sense. Instead we have taken particular case studies as exemplary of these broader themes.

In part I, "Tissue Banks: Managing the Tissue Economy," we focus on the place of tissue banks in developing and circulating tissue economies, particularly how they must now adjudicate between the ontological and communal values associated with gratuitous donation, and the market values introduced by the growing role of biocommercial enterprise in developing tissue-based therapies. In chapter 1 we examine the fate of blood economies since Titmuss's analysis, focusing particularly on the HIV and hepatitis C contamination scandals of the 1980s, and we discuss the decisive role played by blood banks and their understandings of the gift-commodity relation in these scandals. This history is by now well documented (Starr 1998; Rabinow 1999;

Bayer 1999), and we draw on this material as a necessary introduction to the contemporary political economy of human tissues. However, we also use this history to illustrate the inauguration of a new kind of tissue economy, the autologous economy. Here the donors use the regenerative powers of their own bodies for themselves rather than for others, and use the tissue bank not as a point of redistribution but as a place to set up private tissue accounts to save their tissues for the future. This emergence of the autologous tissue economy is taken up again in chapter 4 in relation to umbilical cord blood and regenerative medicine.

In chapter 2 we examine the creation of a new kind of tissue bank, the UK Stem Cell Bank, which has an explicit remit to facilitate the donation of embryos by demonstrating good governance of the human stem cell economy. Embryos are particularly problematic forms of human tissue, because they are heavily charged with local, ontological significance yet form the starting point for complex, global flows through for-profit biotechnology circuits, with highly uncertain therapeutic outcomes and destinations. We argue that the UK Stem Cell Bank is a highly strategic initiative, set up to manage at least some strands of these global flows in accordance with ideas of both national and public good, and to mange potential conflicts of interest between donors, commercial actors, and (eventual) recipients.

Part II, "Waste and Tissue Economies," moves from the highly ontologized tissues described in part I to an examination of waste tissues in the organization of tissue economies. Waste, as a source of latent value, is essential to all forms of economy. While much of the force of Titmuss's account depended upon his demonstration that the market system of blood collection in the United States wasted far more blood than the British gift system, he understood "waste" as an entirely negative category, simply a loss of value. Waste as a source of positive value is a possibility unexamined by Titmuss, and one absent from his theory of tissue economies. We investigate the ways that designating some tissues as "hospital waste" severs them from the identity of their (often-unwitting) donors and frees them up for innovative and profitable forms of circulation and transformation. In chapter 3 we revisit a legal case with a now extensive commentary literature, *Moore v. Regents of the University of California,* in which a U.S.

citizen, John Moore, tries and fails to establish property rights in a patented cell line established without his consent from his spleen tissues. Our task in revisiting this case is to elucidate the central role that designations of waste played in the ruling, and play more generally in the circulation of human tissues through for-profit laboratories. Moore's case makes plain that the designation of some tissues as waste, as valueless or dangerous before their entry point into the revivifying space of biocommerce, is a crucial move in securing the intellectual property rights and profit margins of the biotechnology industry.

In chapter 4 we examine another transformation of waste into positive value, that of umbilical cord blood. In the late 1980s cord blood was dramatically revalued, from (useful) detritus to precious therapeutic substance, a treatment for life-threatening blood disorders in children. At this point it became a part of two distinct systems of value: a redistributive gift economy, in which public cord-blood banks accept allogenic donations and store cord blood to be matched with a needy recipient in the future; and a private, autologous cord-blood system, in which parents open a personal cord-blood account for their child, for future use. This second system of value gives eloquent expression, we suggest, to both the neoliberal appeal of investing a part of the body in the future and the increasingly important regenerative models of tissue economy, in which each person relies not on the surpluses generated by another body but on the regenerative possibilities of his or her own body.

Part III, "Biogifts of Capital," examines situations where the social virtues historically associated with gift economies are claimed by advocates of various kinds of tissue markets. Chapter 5 examines several cases in which commodified tissues have functioned as the basis for kinds of civil belonging and public circulation. It looks in particular at the paradoxical status of biotechnology patents. One the one hand, these can be configured as a form of exclusive property right, enclosing what might otherwise be public domain knowledge or low-cost biomaterials within the high walls of maximum license fees and stringent boundary policing. On the other, legal devices like the General Public License and public good considerations in the pricing of license fees allow many patent holders to favor some form of biomedical "commons," where knowledge, tissues, and techniques can circulate under conditions of common access and contribution. At the same time, some patient groups have entered into exclusive patent-based relationships with medical researchers, co-managing access to the knowledge and profits generated from research on their tissue fragments. As medical charities and patient advocacy groups become powerful players in funding and directing for-profit therapeutic research, these kinds of arrangements seem set to become more common.

Chapter 6 examines the practices and arguments around organ markets. National gift economies in cadaveric organs have proved unable to meet the demand for transplants, and waiting lists for organs grow ever longer in industrialized nations. We discuss the relationship between these waiting lists and the growth of a global black market in "spare" kidneys, sold by the poor in the South to organ brokers who arrange their transport to wealthy transplant patients. Health economists and some bioethicists regard this black market as the result of the intrinsic inefficiency of gift systems, and advocate the creation of regulated organ markets to undercut the exploitative nature of black markets. We consider the systematic blindness in these arguments to the insatiable nature of demand for transplant organs, driven by the elaboration in both transplant medicine and regenerative medicine of an idea of a regenerative body, whose every loss can be repaired.

This book is ultimately about how the human body's productivity is sutured into social systems of productivity, community, and politics, the various proposals for altering the present arrangements, and the kinds of cultural significance that these proposals carry. In this sense the book is profoundly concerned with the contemporary power relations of life and the life sciences, the sphere of biopolitics (Foucault 1980), and the ways that these power relations frame the domain of bioethics and public policy. The capacity of commercial biotechnology to generate novel capacities and forms of profit from in vitro human tissues has dramatically transformed these power relations and now, it seems to us, a great deal is at stake in different proposals for the best way to organize tissue economies. We hope that this book contributes significantly to the debate.

PART I

Tissue Banks

MANAGING THE

TISSUE ECONOMY

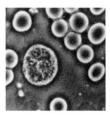 In what sense can we talk about human "tissue economies"? The term implies that tissues have a productivity capable of being ordered in different ways. The celebrated work on biopolitics by Foucault (1980) describes how early modern human bodies, their sexual productivity and labor power, were mobilized both for and against institutions, for and against capital. Here we consider how the medical and biotechnological advances of the late twentieth century mobilize the in vitro productivity of human tissues, their capacities once removed from the body. Within the body, tissues constitute the biological substrate of the self, the condition of viable human life. Once donated, they can sustain the life and health of another. A tissue economy, in our terms, is a system for maximizing this productivity, through strategies of circulation, leverage, diversification, and recuperation. An economy is also a system for adjudicating value (Bourdieu 1984); thus a tissue economy involves hierarchizing the values associated with tissue productivity. As Titmuss's work and our previous discussion suggest, these values are complex and overdetermined—blood for Titmuss has an ontological value, in that it refers to the identity and generosity of the donor. It has use value—it can confer health and indeed save the lives of pa-

tients in need of transfusion. It can be used to constitute social values, creating surpluses of trust, inclusion, and equity among citizens. It has a commodity value, that of an exchangeable object with a price, which can be bought and sold on a market. All of these values remain implicit and potential until they are ordered into an economy. Different forms of circulation (giving, lending, buying) constitute and hierarchize these values of blood in different ways, and produce different social, ethical, and health outcomes.

The biology of the organism involves a complex form of tissue economy, an ordering and coordination of the cells, muscles, organs, and blood, with their different qualities and capacities. The economy of donated tissues is necessarily delimited by this biology. A key feature of tissue economies, as we use this term, is their *technicity*. That is, their overall shape is described at the intersection of the material qualities of tissues—their location and function in the body, their durability, their immunological specificity—with the kinds of technology available to procure, potentiate, store, and distribute them. At the micro-social level, some tissues, for example solid organs, offer little affordance to technical intervention: they are transferred between donor and recipient bodies intact, in a more or less "native" state. Their productivity is strictly in vivo, not amenable to complex technical ordering—though as Hogle (1999) notes, donors themselves may be heavily "processed" before their organs are retrieved to maximize the chances for a successful transplant. Other tissues are open to the micro-technical manipulation of productivity, the maximizing of what Waldby (2000, 2002a) has described elsewhere as "biovalue." This is the surplus of in vitro vitality produced by the biotechnical reformulation of living processes. These tissues can be leveraged biotechnically so that they become more prolific or useful, through processes like the fractioning of blood, the use of polymerase chain reaction (PCR) to amplify genetic sequences, the creation of cell lines, genetic engineering, and cell nuclear transfer. A great deal of medical biotechnology is devoted to this amplification or modification of the biological capacities of tissue fragments. Biotechnical procedures induce the tissue fragment to expand, to accelerate or slow cellular processes, to unfurl or recapacitate, to produce new substances or develop along new pathways, to recombine with other fragments and swap properties. This biovaluable engineering is often associated with the requirements for patent, so that surplus in vitro vitality may eventually be transformed into surplus commercial profits, as well as in vivo therapies. In this way, the productivity of tissues intersects with the productivity of markets, entering into the circuits of national and transnational capital economies.

At the macro-social level, tissues circulate through the social body according to technical principles that regulate their accumulation, transformation, multiplication, distribution, and utilization. Different tissues exist under different conditions of scarcity and demand, fragility and robustness. Some can be cryopreserved for long periods, others rapidly lose their efficacy in storage. Some travel well through space, others suffer. Human tissues require varying forms of social triage and technical expertise in harvesting, storage, transportation, and transplant to ensure that their productivity is maximized. Unlike genetic information, which can be stored and manipulated in the durable form of computer data, therapeutic tissues are an exhaustible resource, whose value or utility could be lost with poor management (Laurie 2001). They require marshalling and oversight, economy in the archaic sense of "husbandry."

These technical matters are never socially neutral, however. Considerations of harvesting, biovaluable engineering, storage, and distribution are also political considerations. Economies, as Marx knew and as Titmuss reminds us, are always forms of social relationship. Different forms of economic exchange constitute the social fabric in different ways. Economies are, to use Michel Callon's term, "social networks," and entities that are traded or circulated through economies are "caught up in a network of relations, in a flow of intermediaries which circulate, connect, link and reconstitute identities" (Callon 1998, 17). As we discussed in the Introduction, tissue economies are analyzed predominantly in terms of a gift-commodity dichotomy, which we believe oversimplifies the complex terrain of contemporary tissue economies. However, we would retain the wider point made in these analyses: the forms of circulation characteristic of any particular tissue economy both presuppose and constitute certain kinds of social relations, and indeed power relations. In this sense the circulation of tissues constitutes a *political economy*. All systems of value are implicated in a politics, Appadurai (1986) argues, "in the broad sense of relations, assumptions, and contests pertaining to power": "[The most ordinary exchanges] would not be possible were it not for a broad set of agreements concerning what is desirable, what a reasonable 'exchange of sacrifices' comprises, and who is permitted to exercise what kind of effective demand in what circumstances. . . . Not all parties share the same interests in any specific regime of value, nor are the interests of any two parties in a given exchange identical" (Appadurai 1986, 57).

We shall see in the following chapters that human tissue economies are sites for precisely this kind of contestation. The values attributed to human tissues are always contingent on the particular cultural, ontological, epistemological, and historical significance that they have for different actors in the various tissue economies: donors, recipients, family members, medical staff, venture capitalists, and so on. Hence these values are complex and contested—in part because the social and technical trajectories of tissues are themselves so complex. Tissues that move from bodies to tissue banks to laboratories to other bodies *bring with them* variously ontological values around identity, affective values around kinship, aging, and death, belief systems and ethical standards, and epistemological values and systems of research prestige, as well as use values and exchange values. This overdetermination of the significance of tissues often leads to conflicts and compromises over which system of values will have the upper hand in the way the tissues are harvested, managed, and deployed. The perceived distinction between gift and market systems as a means for harvesting and distribution is frequently expressive of these underlying conflicts.

In the two chapters that follow, we will consider how a particularly important institution in the tissue economy—the tissue bank—is involved in managing these kinds of conflicts around the various regimes of value implicated in two different tissue economies—blood and human embryonic stem cells.

1

Blood Banks, Risk,

and Autologous Donation

THE GIFT OF BLOOD TO ONESELF

Tissue Banks As the name implies, tissue banks are central institutions in regulating various tissue economies. These institutions solicit tissues from donor populations or medical intermediaries (clinics, pathology laboratories), accumulate and process them in various ways, and redistribute them for research or therapeutic applications. Some aspects of contemporary tissue banking have their origins in the nineteenth-century medical museum, established to collect normal and pathological biological specimens—organs, tumours, skeletons, fetuses—for purposes of medical education and anatomical studies. As medical interest shifted in the twentieth century from gross anatomy to the body's biochemistry and cellular structure, such collections of organs were displaced by tissue samples, used to research particular medical conditions or epidemiological trends in populations (Lawrence 1998). With the creation of the first blood depots between the world wars, tissue banks also became places where tissue could be moved from body to body as therapy.

The term "tissue bank" encompasses a wide range of biomedical practices and functions. The Nuffield Report on ethical and legal issues in human tissue management in the United Kingdom summarizes the different kinds of tissue banks: "The term tissue bank encompasses both institutions that handle primarily fresh tissue and those that maintain collections of preserved tissue. . . . There is also a distinction to be drawn between banks that supply tissue primarily for therapy, and those that supply it for research purposes. . . . Finally, tissue banks may operate simply as central stores, providing research workers or surgeons with access to certain tissue, or those who organise them may pursue a more active policy of organising collection and distribution" (Hurley 1995, 29).

Unlike genetic databases, which are primarily concerned with managing genetic information derived from tissue samples, tissue banks are concerned with the storage, research, and therapeutic applications of the "wet" biological material itself, rather than sequence information abstracted from the material. Tissue banks may be public, national institutions, like the National Blood Service (NBS) in the United Kingdom, or for-profit enterprises like the private umbilical-cord-blood companies now starting up around the world (see chapter 4). Virtually every organ and tissue type in the body has its cognate tissue bank, and citizens in industrial nations are more and more likely to have some fragment of their body retained in a tissue bank: "There are now brain tissue banks, breast tissue banks, blood banks, umbilical cord banks, sperm banks, and tissue repositories for studying AIDS, Alzheimer's, mental illnesses, and aging. More than 282 million archived and identifiable pathological specimens from more than 176 million individuals are currently being stored in United States repositories. At least 20 million new specimens are added each year. . . . Virtually everyone has his or her tissue 'on file' somewhere" (Andrews and Nelkin 2001, 4–5).

As the quote from the Nuffield Council Report states, tissue banks may exist primarily for research purposes or for therapy, or they may combine these functions. Therapeutic tissue banks are those that transfer tissues from donors to recipients, rather than from donor to laboratory as research-oriented banks do. The most familiar and oldest of these is the blood bank, first termed "bank" by Bernard Fantus, an American physician who was among the early developers of systems of blood storage. "Noting the process involved deposits and withdrawals, he came up with a name for the facility: blood bank" (Starr 2001, 120). Several other kinds of tissues can be banked for therapeutic or reproductive purposes. Skin can be donated posthumously, or after surgery, stored for up to three years, and used for burn treatments. Bone can be procured during hip replacements, stored for up to five years, and used for limb reconstruction or treatment after bone cancer. Heart valves and corneas can be banked (Hurley 1995). Sperm and embryos can be donated, frozen, and used later for reproduction. Umbilical-cord blood is increasingly harvested during birth, banked, and used to treat blood disorders. Human embryonic and adult stem cells can also be banked, and the next chapter will examine the UK Stem Cell Bank, the first national public stem cell bank in the world, in some detail.

Each of these institutions is the site for accumulating valuable tissues, but as we discussed above, the value of human tissue is complex and overdetermined by considerations of ontological status, clinical efficacy, knowledge production, social relationships, and market forces. The management of tissue banks may involve mediating between conflicting demands arising from these values. Tissue banks may find themselves abruptly enmeshed in a complex biopolitical field. Recent events at the Alder Hey Children's Hospital in Liverpool are a case in point. In common with many other hospitals, Alder Hey harvested organs during postmortems, and over a number of years built up a large collection of tissue for research and teaching. Most of the parents of children who had died in the hospital were unaware that a postmortem had taken place or that organs had been retained, because they had not been asked for formal consent. In 1999 a community health director, concerned that the lack of formal consent contravened the Human Tissue Act and the rights of parents, made the existence of this collection public. Moreover, the hospital did not have an active research program that used the tissues, so their retention appeared somewhat gratuitous. This revelation caused a scandal and led to an independent inquiry in 2000 into "the removal, retention and disposal of human organs and tissues following post mortem examination at Alder Hey" (Royal Liverpool Children's Inquiry 2001, 5). Parents who were informed of the practice as part of the inquiry or through media coverage reacted with grief and anger. Some stated that they felt as though the hospital had robbed them of their child, violated their trust, and exploited them at their most vulnerable moments. Many parents and relatives demanded possession of the retained organs and held second funerals, stating that they felt as if their child had died all over again (Royal Liverpool Children's Inquiry 2001).

Here we can see that a paternalistic, medically driven approach to the collection of tissues has failed in the task of managing the different meanings and values that tissues have for the various parties involved. For medical researchers, retained organs have primarily epistemological and pedagogical value, a value somewhat neglected in the Alder Hey case. For grieving parents, retained organs are signifiers of their dead child, objects of loss and mourning. Their unauthorized harvesting and retention is a violation of both the child's body and their rights as parents to control the disposal of that body in a loving and dignified way. The hospital had failed to modify its procedures in line with the general move toward better enforcement of the rights of patients and exhaustive use of consent procedures recommended in a range of inquiries and reports produced in the United Kingdom throughout the 1990s.[1] These reports in turn reflect changes in public attitudes about medical treatment of the human body, including, as we have already described to some extent, a strengthening human rights discourse around biomedicine and the respect owed to human bodies, and increased awareness of the commercial and health value of tissues and organs (Laurie 2001). These changes have increased the complexity of values that tissue banks and collections like those at Alder Hey hospital must try to manage. In response to the Alder Hey events, a new body of legislation, the Human Tissue Act 2004, has been introduced in Parliament to strengthen the requirements for consent where tissue is removed from the deceased.

Blood Banking   In this chapter we focus on one kind of human tissue—peripheral blood, the blood which circulates throughout the body, in contradistinction to umbilical cord blood, which is discussed in chapter 4. Therefore this chapter follows on from our analysis of blood banking begun in the Introduction. We will first discuss the ways that blood banking developed in the years following Titmuss's study, and the implications that these developments have for his analysis. As we have seen, Titmuss argued that an exclusive reliance on a gift economy for blood was a strategy inherently able to manage in a nonconflicting way the various values attributed to blood. It would ensure a clean supply, protect the dignity of both donor and recipient, promote positive, inclusive social relationships, and distribute blood equitably from those who could afford to give to those in need, irrespective of ability to pay. We will consider how this strategy failed to reconcile the interests of donors and recipients, and the values of good citizenship and public health, in the wake of changing demands attendant on new treatments and the rapid globalization of the blood supply. We will also consider the rise of a new kind of gift economy for blood, the autologous donation, or the donation of blood to oneself. We will argue that this autologous economy is a response to the blood bank's ongoing difficulties in harmonizing competing interests and values. While we will focus primarily on Britain, we will also draw on developments in the United States and France.

At the time Titmuss wrote *The Gift Relationship*, the ontological and civil status of blood donation was more straightforward in some important respects than it is today. There were two technical features of blood that contributed to its being theorized as a gift circulated between citizens. First, as we have already noted, blood was primarily transfused as whole blood. In Britain in 1975, six years after Titmuss's study was published, 90 percent of all transfusions were of whole blood (Martlew 1997). That is, the donor's blood was transferred in a single unit, in a stable form and composition, to a recipient. The National Blood Service (NBS), with a system of transfusion centers and subsidiary blood banks, acted as a storage and transfer point between a specific donor and a specific patient, although the identity of each remained unknown to the other. The bank itself made some technical interventions in the transferred substance: it added citrate to stop clotting, refrigerated the blood to slow deterioration, and ensured that handling conditions were sanitary to prevent contamination. It then distributed blood to hospitals for transfusion. So the NBS effectively acted as the collection and distribution point for units of blood that remained in a relatively stable form throughout the process, from point of donation to point of transfusion.

We suggest that this relative stability of the tissue transferred lent itself to Titmuss's theorizing of blood donation as the exchange of gifts between particular, though anonymous, persons. To some extent, the transfer of whole blood resembles the economy of contemporary organ donation: it is one-to-one, it transfers a stable entity that has had little medical alteration, it is nonreversible, and the recipient cannot generally repay the gift that is given. Several studies (Fox and Swazey 1992; Lock 2002; Rosengarten 2001) confirm that the organ recipient experiences this kind of tissue economy as highly personal. Transplant patients feel that "part of the donor's self or personhood has been transmitted along with the organ" (Fox and Swazey 1992, 36). Lock (2002) observes that it is common for organ recipients to worry about the gender, ethnicity, skin color, personality, and social status of their donors, and be concerned that the organ's "identity" may overtake them. The analogy with organ donation is admittedly imperfect: whole organs cannot be banked, so they must be transferred from donor to recipient in real time; whole organ donation is generally posthumous; and organs can only be given once, whereas blood is a renewable substance. The same person can donate repeatedly without great risk to his or her health. For these reasons whole organs have a greater aura of singularity and sacrifice than blood does, and seem likely to carry a greater ontological charge than a blood donation. Nevertheless, we would argue that the kind of whole blood transfusion assumed by Titmuss, in its simple, one-to-one ratio, lends itself to the specification of blood as an act of exchange between identifiable subjects. The blood given retains a relatively stable relationship to the donor—it designates a specifiable fraction of a particular person's body, and is incorporated in that ratio by another, particular person. Here the blood bank is understood to play a transparent role, simply facilitating the exchange without fundamentally altering its nature.

The second technical feature of blood banking at that time was its spatial limitations. Whole blood is a relatively fragile substance. It requires stringent conditions of sterilization, refrigeration, and handling to preserve its vital qualities. It is not readily transported across long distances. As Starr (1998) notes, this fragility had presented particular difficulties in the Allied war effort. The U.S. military was unable to transport whole blood to the front because it deteriorated too rapidly to endure shipment. Instead they shipped plasma (a more durable fraction of blood, without red blood cells), used to prevent shock. Plasma can keep for several months, does not require tissue typing, and can endure rough handling, and thus it lent itself to international export, although it proved less effective than whole blood in restoring health. The fragility of whole blood meant that after the war, civilian blood systems were nationally based and regionally organized. Initially nation-states did not export or import blood, but only collected it within the boundaries of national space.[2] Hence the circulation of blood was readily conceptualized as part of the creation of horizontal, equitable relationships of national solidarity among citizens, and between citizens and the state.

In summary, the spatial limits of the whole blood economy were also the limits of the nation, and blood banks were primarily points for the exchange of whole blood units between one person and another. These two features of the blood supply in the late 1960s facilitated Titmuss's theorization of blood donation as a gift between citizens, a form of civil intersubjectivity and intercorporeality (Weiss 1999). However, within fifteen years of the publication of *The Gift Relationship*, the technical conditions of blood, the possibilities for its processing, circulation, and incorporation, had become quite different. The ratios of donation to transfusion and other kinds of incorporation (notably the self-administration of coagulant agents by hemophiliacs) changed dramatically, so that one-to-one donation was now the exception. At the same time, the kinds of space through which blood could travel had expanded and complicated dramatically. A burgeoning, transnational pharmaceutical industry played a crucial role in the commercial development of these changes, and in their strategic exploitation. These transformations and their consequences, discussed below, have helped to reconfigure the significance of the blood supply. It is now commonly regarded not as a distributor of health and a benevolent mediator between fellow citizens, but as a distributor of risk and illness and a dangerous mediator between clean and infected sectors of the population.

Fractionation and the Globalization of the Blood Supply   Today whole blood transfusion is rare. In 1996 less than 5 percent of all transfusions in the United Kingdom were of whole blood (Martlew 1997). Most blood is transfused as fractions, subsets of blood proteins tailored to suit the clinical needs of the particular patient's condition. The fractioning of blood began during the Second World War, when the success of plasma encouraged biochemists in the United States to research other possible ways to break blood down into its components. Several fractions were isolated from liquid plasma during or soon after the war: fibrinogen, or clotting factor; a variety of gamma globulins, or antibodies, used to make vaccines; albumin, used as part of anti-shock therapy; anti-Rh factor, used in treating Rh+ babies born to Rh− mothers; and reagents useful for some laboratory tests. Plasma and albumin were not retained in a liquid form but freeze-dried, to be reconstituted at the point of transfusion. By 1950 the nonplasma components of whole blood could also be isolated into red cells, white cells, and platelets.

This isolation of blood proteins meant that blood could be used in much more flexible, strategic, and clinically targeted ways than whole blood. Unlike in the one-to-one economy dictated by the use of whole blood, a single blood donation could be broken down into its components and used by several patients. Starr (1998) reports that the biochemists in the United States involved in blood fractioning described it precisely as "blood economy," a system for the leveraging of the value of each unit of whole blood. He cites a description of "blood economy" provided by Charles Janeway, a biochemist involved in the early fractioning work: "Normally, [Janeway wrote,] if you collect four units of blood you can treat four individuals, assuming they need only one unit each. But if you first separate the liquid into red cells and plasma, you can then treat six individuals—four with the red cells and two with the plasma . . . You can increase the blood's usefulness again if you first fractionate the plasma into albumin, gamma globulin, [and other components]. In this way you can treat a total of twenty-three people—all with the original four units" (Starr 1998, 178).

In Britain these techniques were not used at first, and whole blood donation continued for many years. Martlew (1997) observes that blood fractioning could only become a standard procedure in Britain once the NBS moved in 1975 from its old collection system of reusable glass bottles to a modular system of polymer containers, airtight tubes, and incorporated syringes, which allowed differential collection and storage conditions. The development of aphaeresis donation, or plasmapheresis as it is termed in the United States, also facilitated the greater use of fractioned blood. In aphaeresis the donor does not give whole blood. Instead the blood circulates through a centrifuge, the plasma component is separated out, and the red blood cells are re-infused in the donor. Aphaeresis made plasma much more readily available than whole-blood donation, and so increased the volume of plasma-fractioned products in use. Patients became less likely to receive blood in the same form in which it was donated, and more likely to receive an increasingly processed fraction of a donation, or several fractions of several donations. The ratios involved in the blood economy had fundamentally altered.

Another major alteration to the donor-recipient ratio occurred in the area of hemophilia treatment.[3] The fractioning of plasma allowed hemophiliacs to keep frozen plasma, which contained the absent clotting factor, at home for self-infusion. In 1965 biochemists in the United States produced a concentrate of clotting factor, cryoprecipitate, which could be kept frozen at home, and a few years later a far more concentrated form of clotting factor, Factor VIII, was developed. Factor VIII is a powder, which can be reconstituted in water and injected, rapidly stopping an incipient bleed. This development represented a major advance in hemophilia health, longevity, and quality of life. The life expectancy of hemophiliacs doubled between 1968 and 1979 (Rabinow 1999). Factor VIII was a highly concentrated substance, however, and required the processing of large quantities of plasma. The pharmaceutical companies producing Factor VIII in the United States derived it by pooling plasma from often thousands of donors, a practice that guaranteed the hepatitis contamination of almost all pools. A hemophiliac administering a single dose of Factor VIII might incorporate fractions of thousands of bodies, and the related hepatitis risk, with a single injection. While other plasma products could be sterilized with heat treatment, clotting factor was understood to be destroyed by heat.

This series of technological innovations made donated blood much more of a mediated substance than that described by Titmuss. The N BS no longer simply offered a way to move blood from one body into another but played a more complex role in leveraging the usefulness of each donation by splitting and processing it into multiple products with varying destinations. In the process it maximized the use value of the donation but also diluted its ontological and civil value, making it more like a pharmaceutical substance and less like a gift from one citizen to another.

The second important change in the organization of the blood supply, its internationalization, was a response to the escalation of demand for blood and plasma products as new treatments were developed. The production of Factor VIII and other blood concentrates required very large quantities of blood. The demand for whole blood and cell-based blood products also increased throughout the 1970s with the development of certain types of surgery—hip and organ replacements, open heart surgery—and cancer treatments that produced anemia as a side effect (Martlew 1997). While Britain could still provide its own supplies of whole blood, it could not recruit sufficient voluntary donors to meet the national demand for plasma products. Like most of western Europe, Britain did not use plasmapheresis donation. The lengthy donation times and the pain of the procedure made it very difficult to recruit voluntary donors, and the idea of using paid donors was an affront to the British ethos of the gift relationship. Instead plasma was spun off from whole-blood donations. Self-sufficiency in national blood supply was a policy target throughout the 1970s, but the Elstree Blood Products Laboratory, which produced Factor VIII, found that it could only supply 20 percent of demand, because plasma donations were insufficient (Berridge 1996).

To meet the demand for Factor VIII, the United Kingdom, in common with France, Holland, and Switzerland, turned to the international trade in plasma managed by pharmaceutical companies, precisely the companies criticized by Titmuss in his study. These companies maintained paid plasma collection programs, at first among the urban poor in the United States. However, the demand for plasma was such that these companies turned to offshore supplies, purchased from facilities based in Latin America, Africa, and the Caribbean, which recruited paid donors from among local populations. So while whole-blood collection remained under the control of nation-states, working as a gift system among national citizens, plasma became a global commodity, sold by the poor of the developing world and the United States to the citizens of western Europe, with pharmaceutical companies based in the United States acting as brokers. By the late

1970s these companies supplied approximately half of western Europe's plasma needs. As Starr puts it, the United States acted as the "OPEC of plasma, exporting plasma and its derivatives throughout the world" (Starr 2001, 120–21).

The nations of western Europe were unable to sequester their gift systems from the pressures of an international blood market. Britain sourced half of its Factor VIII supplies from this market by the late 1970s (Berridge 1996). As Berridge puts it, "A 'volunteer image' fronted systems which had become highly dependant on commercial sources. Whereas the blood donation side of the transfusion service dealing in 'whole blood' was volunteer-based in the classic way, blood products were primarily commercial in origin, part of a huge international trade in blood" (Berridge 1996, 38).

HIV, Hepatitis C, and the Legitimation Crisis of the Blood Services   We can see that the image of gifts between citizens within national boundaries conjured by Titmuss was now greatly complicated by the introduction of far more promiscuous, multiple, commodified, and globalized kinds of bodily exchange. Starr summarizes the health risks associated with this situation: "By the late 1970s, the blood-services complex [in the United States] had become an interlocking network that mingled the blood and plasma of millions of people who lived in regions thousands of miles apart. Generally this intermingling proved beneficial: more people received life-saving blood products than ever before. But the distribution also bore peril. Integrating the world's blood products network did more than increase the efficiency of supply—it established optimum conditions for the spread of emerging viruses" (Starr 1998, 265).

Various national blood systems thus came into temporary, serial, or more permanent contact with international commercial systems over which they had no policy or quality control, producing highly complex and unpredictable synergies and unanticipated risks. The international blood complex had become a way to transport and amplify infection risk, moving it around the world, from the bodies of the few to the many through the pooling of plasma and the creation of unsterilized concentrates. The result of these arrangements is now well known. Hemophiliacs, the group with the greatest exposure to these new ratios and global flows, were among the first to develop the symptoms of the disease eventually termed acquired immunodeficiency syndrome (AIDS). Throughout 1982, at the same time as some gay men were exhibiting symptoms of a mysterious new illness, the U.S. Centers for Disease Control (CDC) identified a handful of hemophiliacs with a similar symptom profile—signs of acute immune deficiency and the development of Pneumocystis carinii pneumonia (Waldby 1996). Initially the CDC suspicions that AIDS was blood-borne and represented a threat to the blood supply went largely unheeded.[4] The etiology of AIDS was heavily disputed—initial theories included possible "lifestyle" causes like recreational use of amyl nitrate by gay men or the purported immunosuppressive effects of too much anal sex (Waldby 1996). Hemophilia organizations, after years of advocacy for Factor VIII and tolerance of its hepatitis risks, were initially reluctant to consider the AIDS danger that it might pose, or to recommend a return to safer alternatives like cryoprecipitate, produced in smaller plasma batches (Bayer 1999).

In 1983 the first symptoms of AIDS emerged among hemophiliacs in the United Kingdom. Only at this point did hemophiliacs and others discover that some Factor VIII was sourced from plasma centers in the developing world. Dr. Peter Jones, the director of the Newcastle Hemophilia Center, proved against the denials of the chief medical officer that Factor VIII used by British hemophiliacs was sourced from a company that relied on plasmapheresis centers in Lesotho and Mexico (Berridge 1996). The subsequent debates in Britain about the best way to protect hemophiliacs betrayed a continued tendency to overestimate the efficacy of the national gift system to protect public health. The plasma companies based in the United States reacted to the contamination scares with a rapid research program in ways to sterilize Factor VIII. Early in 1984 they developed a heat treatment process that effectively sterilized it against hepatitis. They hoped that the process might also kill the agent causing AIDS, although it was several months before this could be conclusively proved (Starr 1998). At this point British hematologists had a choice between the commercially produced yet heat-treated Factor VIII, and domestically supplied yet untreated concentrate. As one hematologist commented, "There was a terrible period from the end of 1984 until October 1985 . . . Here we knew the epidemic was very small and we had a policy of educating people and turning people away. . . . The pool was thought to be safe. . . . Our problem was—did you give US stuff where the pool was terrible or unheated British stuff from a safe donor pool. We gave at least two people unheated British stuff and they became infected. We didn't know that an unsafe pool was rendered safe by heating" (Berridge 1996, 47).

By 1983 blood services staff in the United States and Britain generally accepted that AIDS was transmitted through the blood supply, but many argued that the overall risk to recipients was low. As Healy (1999) notes, these claims were based not on any formal statistical risk assessment but on a reluctance to question the quality of donors' blood. In the United States epidemiologists advocated stringent measures to screen donors. In the absence of an AIDS test (not developed until 1985) they suggested using detailed questionnaires to identify male donors who had had sex with men, and a surrogate marker test, the hepatitis B core antibody test, to identify past hepatitis B infection. They argued that the epidemiological similarities between hepatitis B and AIDS made this test useful in screening donors (Bayer 1999).

However in the United States, Britain, France, and elsewhere these measures were repeatedly rejected. The first impulse of the blood services was to protect their donors from embarrassment and trauma, rather than take what they considered extreme measures to secure the safety of the blood supply. In the United States blood banks were unwilling to bear the cost of the hepatitis test, particularly as it was not specific to AIDS infection, and feared that it might lead to blood shortages (Bayer 1999). Gay organizations, only recently legitimate and anxious about their newly won legal status, protested that donor screening would amount to simple homophobia, reminiscent of the laws that for many years in the United States divided black blood from white blood (Shilts 1987). The National Gay Task Force stated that it would educate gay men about the risks of donation but would not endorse the legal exclusion of gay men from donor panels. The blood bank organizations adopted measures that included autologous donation, educating donors, and discreetly discouraging donations from high-risk groups (Starr 1998).

In contrast, the plasma companies, partly in response to lobbying from the hemophilia associations and partly as a way to secure their continued dominance of the international market, immediately adopted an active policy of screening and excluding gay men, Haitians, intravenous drug users, and others considered high risk (Healy 1999). They did not reduce the size of their plasma pools, however, a measure that would have greatly increased the safety but also the processing costs of Factor VIII (Starr 1998). Despite being put in place rapidly, these measures were too late to prevent the majority of hemophiliac infections. By early 1983, when the CDC began its first vigorous advocacy of screening and safety measures, between 62 percent and 89 percent of total hemophiliac infections had already occurred (Korner, Rosenberg, Aledort, et al. 1994).

In France, eventually the locus of the worst AIDS contamination scandal in the developed world,[5] faith in the power of the gift system was at its highest. This faith had a particularly detrimental effect on the assessment of the AIDS risk to the blood supply. On the one hand, AIDS was considered a product of the commercial system in the United States, the system against which the French philosophy of benevolence had always defined itself and from which it considered itself immune. On the other hand, Rabinow (1999) asserts, the right of the donor to give blood was considered sacred. Attempts by the director of the Centre National de Transfusion Sanguine to introduce questionnaires for donors were met by accusations of human rights violations from the press and from gay and human rights groups. As Rabinow comments, "the proverbial heart of the system was the donors. The quality of the blood they gave was secondary to the manner in which they gave it" (Rabinow 1999, 88). In this climate, French blood-banking officials were particularly resistant to any screening procedures. By 1985 only half of blood banks were using any procedures at all to discourage high-risk donors. Moreover, the Centre National continued to distribute non-heat-treated Factor VIII for several months after treated product was available, and to solicit donations from prisoners, a practice by now discontinued throughout the rest of the world. "An excess of faith in the government's blood system and the purity of 'benevolent' donors had set the stage for the spread of AIDS through the French blood system" (Starr 1998, 289).

In Britain the directors of the national blood services decided against asking donors directly about their sexual practices. Instead they produced a discreet explanatory leaflet, to discourage possibly infected donors from giving blood. When Abbott Laboratories, based in the United States, developed the ELISA test for detecting HIV in 1985, the NBS was initially reluctant to use it, fearing that it would deter potential donors and that the tendency for the test to produce false positives would have devastating effects on donors falsely diagnosed. The Department of Health and Social Security held up approval for the test for five months, ostensibly to monitor the performance of the tests in the United States. The delay also allowed the British pharmaceutical company Wellcome to produce a diagnostic kit, eventually approved by the department for use in the United Kingdom (Berridge 1996).

The Limits of the Gift Relationship   The contamination of blood and blood products during the 1980s made visible the latent tensions and limits of the gift economy. First, as Rabinow observes, "the limits of any 'national' system were underscored by the growing internationalism of markets for blood products" (Rabinow 1999, 72). Throughout the 1970s and 1980s blood became a more mobile, flexible, and specialized substance, needed for more and more kinds of treatment. It also became a global commodity brokered by international pharmaceutical companies, as demand in the North expanded and supply in the South became better organized. These developments placed insupportable pressure on nationally based volunteer systems, effectively destroying the barriers between national and international blood, and between blood that was given and blood that was sold.

Second, AIDS contamination demonstrated the inability of gift systems to guarantee the security of the blood supply. As Healy (1999) points out, the relationship between gift or market systems for blood and contamination risk is a highly contingent one. In the absence of epidemiological information about the distribution of a particular infectious disease, either voluntary or paid suppliers might represent a contamination risk. While "serum hepatitis,"[6] the disease of concern to Titmuss, was concentrated among the poor and indigent paid blood donors in the United States, the epidemiology of HIV was quite different: "In the case of AIDS, a population of responsible, voluntary donors happened to be co-extensive with a large chunk of the disease-bearing population. The blood banks knew homosexual men to be reliable givers and good volunteers. As it turned out, they were also important vectors for HIV. The voluntary system ended up attracting people who contaminated the supply. But, as with commercial donors and hepatitis, they contaminated the supply not because they were donors, but because they had HIV. Titmuss's system ended up selecting the wrong people in much the same way as the previous market arrangement had selected the wrong people: by accident" (Healy 1999, 534).

Third, the AIDS contamination crisis demonstrated the inability of gift systems to harmonize the interests of donors and recipients under all conditions. As we have seen, Titmuss's account asserts that the gift of blood is beyond calculability and power relations, because it is anonymous and therefore lacks the dimension of personal aggrandizement, obligation, and strategy highlighted in Mauss's account of gift economies. Nevertheless, the contamination of the blood supply made evident the asymmetric positions of donor and recipient implicit in the system. For the various national blood services, particularly the western European ones, the donor's sacrifice is the act that creates the various forms of value attributed to banked blood—its use value as a therapeutic substance and its civil value in creating a social surplus. Recipients of transfusions and blood products are simply the recipients of value, its consumers. At a more instrumental level too, blood donors are "relatively rare. Recipients are all too common" (Healy 1999, 541). As the managers of blood's value, the banks believed that it was the donors and their readiness to make this sacrifice that must be protected.[7] Consequently, they were unwilling to introduce screening systems that would distinguish between donors. Rabinow puts it succinctly: "the primary social link is between donors. The link with those who receive the blood is secondary" (Rabinow 1999, 85). Under these circumstances, as we have seen, the gift system did not successfully tie together all the complex values associated with blood. Rather it placed the values of public health and civil generosity at odds with each other, and privileged the latter: "Public health operates under the economy of 'good administration'; one needs to know what resources are available and to take them up as things to be collected, stored, and distributed as efficiently as possible. The economy of the *bénévole* [gift]

system differed: the *'plus,'* its symbolic difference, implied by the benevolent system is respect for human dignity. The blood transfusion
issue was one moment when the two logics of value clashed" (Rabinow 1999, 86). In contrast, the plasma companies, unencumbered
by moral obligations or strong organizational bonds to their paid suppliers, and with an interest in maintaining their markets against competitors, acted quickly to exclude infected suppliers and introduce tests
as they became available (Healy 1999).

In the end, the blood banks' privileging of donors over recipients
contributed to worldwide HIV transmission in significant ways. A
survey of transfusion-related AIDS cases contracted by 1993 found
almost six thousand cases in Europe and over eight thousand in the
United States. France had the highest overall incidence of AIDS related
to transfusion in Europe, with almost as many cases as the United
States despite a much smaller population, and the United Kingdom
had relatively high rates of transmission associated with hemophilia
(Franceschi, Dal Maso, and La Vecchia 1995).

**The Blood of Others: Transfusion, Risk and Public Perceptions of the
Blood Supply**   The contamination of the blood supply in the United
States, the United Kingdom, France, and elsewhere was a trauma
whose repercussions are still playing out in the policies and practices
of blood banks, and in public perceptions about the safety of blood. In
the wake of HIV contamination, and the identification of hepatitis C
contamination in the late 1980s, many members of the population
now regard the banks as inherent sites of infectious risk. "Europeans
and Blood," a public opinion survey conducted by Eurobarometer in
1995 of thirteen thousand residents in the twelve member states of the
European Union, found that 70 percent of respondents were afraid to
receive blood transfusions because of the risk of AIDS; 23 percent of
respondents said that blood transfusions were less safe than they had
been ten years ago, although 55 percent considered them safer. In a
survey of 1,204 people conducted in the United States in 1997 and
1998, almost half the respondents rated the risk of infection from
blood transfusion as moderate or high, and a third said that they
would refuse a blood transfusion from the blood bank (Finucane,
Slovic, and Mertz 2000). The authors suggest that the high levels of

anxiety identified in their study derive from the perception that transfusion has the catastrophic potential to amplify infection, and that the sources of blood are unknown and uncontrollable:

> The main cause of concern for the public stems historically from infection of blood in the 1980s with HIV and Hepatitis C. Such infection signals catastrophe to people, because the HIV and HCV epidemics have seemed relentless, and they have horrific and potentially fatal consequences. The risk with blood is also involuntary: recipients of blood transfusions would typically face death or severe health consequences if the transfusion were not administered, so they have little choice in the matter. Moreover, unless recipients donate their own blood, the blood used in transfusions is perceived to come from an uncontrollable source. That is, blood is contributed by strangers and is stored and distributed by a large "blood bank," neither of which can be influenced very much by an individual patient. (Finucane, Slovic, and Mertz 2000, 1021)

Here we can see that for these respondents, the blood bank has become a distributor not of health and benevolence but of risk and contamination, simply a conduit from one infected body to another. A recent Australian study carried out by Waldby and colleagues (2004) among a sample of ninety-two people found similar understandings of the blood bank. The overwhelming majority of the people interviewed expressed some anxiety about receiving a blood transfusion, and many portrayed the blood bank as simply a conduit of infection between on the one hand "risky" sectors of the population, particularly intravenous drug users, sex workers, and gay men, who are perceived as reservoirs of HIV and hepatitis, and on the other hand "clean" sectors, in which they generally placed themselves. Here we can see an inverted image of Titmuss's gift. The blood bank's systemic and technical mediation of the blood supply is downplayed, treated as a neutral passage point between bodies. However, in this case it distributes the gift not of health but of illness, given not by an altruistic fellow citizen but by a shadowy and treacherous other.

The contamination incidents have also had serious effects on the *donation* of blood. Blood donation in the United States, Britain, and elsewhere has been in decline since 1984 (Robertson and McQueen

1994; Wallace et al. 1995; Wallace et al. 1998; Sullivan et al. 2002). At least some of this decline is due to a public perception that even the donation of blood carries an infection risk.[8] According to a series of surveys carried out in the United Kingdom in the late 1980s, a significant number of respondents believed that HIV could be transmitted to donors as well as transfusion recipients (MacAskill et al. 1989; Nutbeam et al. 1989). More recent studies (Bhopal et al. 1992; Robertson and McQueen 1994) have found that this idea persists, so that in a study by Robertson and McQueen of 17,537 randomly sampled respondents in Scotland, 13 percent of blood donors and 27 percent of nondonors stated that there was a risk of infection from giving blood. The Eurobarometer survey (European Commission 1995) found that medical grounds were the most common reason that respondents cited for not giving blood, closely followed by a fear of contracting AIDS. In Europe as a whole, 35 percent of nondonors cited the fear of AIDS as their major deterrent. It is evident that many people in the developed world consider the blood bank a site of contamination risk, at the points of both donation and transfusion.

Banks have tried to address these fears and rebuild trust among both donors and transfusion recipients through public education campaigns, organizational reform, and above all the adoption of rigorous risk-management and risk-profiling strategies. Donors in the United States, the United Kingdom, and elsewhere endure a battery of questions regarding their sexual practices, history of drug use, tattoos, body piercing, medical history, travel history, and other factors that might point to high risk. Increasingly elaborate testing technology is used to identify pathogens in donated blood. In the early 1980s, at the time of the first HIV infection events, the only mandatory serological tests in Britain were for syphilis and hepatitis B. All blood has been screened for HIV since October 1985, and for hepatitis C since 1991. In 2002 the NBS introduced tests for HTLV (human T-cell lymphotropic virus), which infects white blood cells, and the more sensitive nucleic acid tests for HIV and hepatitis C. British donors whose blood is found to be infected are notified and excluded from the donor panel (Martlew 1997). Blood agencies in Britain are now concerned that variant Creutzfeldt-Jakob disease (vCJD), the human form of bovine spongiform encephalopathy, or "mad cow" disease, usually contracted through the consumption of infected beef products, may have entered the blood supply. At time of writing, the health secretary in the United Kingdom had identified one probable transfusion-related death from vCJD.[9] No test yet exists for vCJD, a problem that has led several countries, including the United States, Canada, and Australia, to exclude residents of the United Kingdom from their donor pools.

In other words, blood banks have tried to rebuild their social contacts with their donors and patients by constructing ever more finely meshed, widely advertised, and expensive methods of risk detection and management. More and more sectors of the potential donor population are excluded, as blood services seek to identify and preempt any possible new source of risk. These policies necessarily produce a vulnerable blood supply, because the source of supply has become increasingly constrained, and anxieties about the safety of donation prevent other eligible donors from coming forward.

In summary, quite large sectors of the population in the United States and Europe mistrust the safety of the blood supply, despite the adoption of extensive risk management, testing, and inventory control measures by blood services. We will now discuss an emerging trend in blood donation that arises from this lack of trust and sense of risk.

Autologous Donation: The Gift to Oneself During the H IV contamination scares of the mid-1980s, one response from both patients and clinicians was a demand for easier access to autologous blood donation. Autologous blood donation is a technique first used successfully in humans in the first decades of the twentieth century, often as a way to transfuse patients with rare blood groups (Nagai 1998). The autologous donor does not give blood anonymously into a general allogenic collection, but instead establishes an individual "account" from which he or she can later draw. A few weeks before an elective surgical procedure, the autologous donor will provide between one and four units of blood. In effect this is not a "donation" of blood but a "deposit," building up a store that can be withdrawn and used if needed. Not all elective patients are eligible for autologous donation—a patient must be in good health to tolerate the preoperative depletion of blood.

Autologous donation was not widely used before the H IV contamination of the blood supply. Physicians realized that this was one technique they could use to protect patients needing nonemergency surgery. Since then autologous donation has become more readily available, although uptake varies markedly from country to country. A recent report by the Council of Europe (2000) found that in 1997 in the United States 8 percent of all blood donated was autologous, whereas the average in the European Union was 4 percent. Within the EU, Germany, Italy, and France were the greatest users of autologous blood, between 6 percent and 9 percent of donations, whereas the Scandinavian countries discouraged it on the grounds that the risk of infection from allogenic blood is very low. The blood services in Britain have also tried to restrict its use to some extent, although recently, in the wake of the vCJD scare, this approach has changed. We discuss the significance of this change below.

Most patients request autologous donation specifically because of their anxieties about contamination of the blood supply. A Canadian study (Graham et al. 1999) of seventy-eight autologous donors found that 56 percent cited the avoidance of HIV, hepatitis, or other blood-borne pathogens as their main reason for pre-donating, while 28 percent stated they felt safer donating their own blood. Another study found that some surgeons advocated autologous donation to their patients as a form of "defensive medicine in response to medico-legal pressures, and to ensure a patient's clean bill in terms of infectious disease" (Treloar et al. 2001, 233). The Eurobarometer survey found that 25 percent of respondents would only accept their own blood in the event of a blood transfusion, while a further 23 percent would only accept blood from a friend or relative. Respondents in the United Kingdom were more trusting of the blood supply than in the EU as a whole, yet even so, 24 percent stated they would only accept their own blood or that of a friend or relative.

In the study carried out by Waldby and colleagues (2004) almost all of the ninety-two respondents expressed a preference for autologous donation if they required a nonemergency transfusion, including the fifteen respondents who were regular blood donors themselves. The six respondents who had actually made autologous donations did so because of fears about the sensitivity of screening procedures and the possibility that an intravenous drug user or person infected with HIV might be the source of the blood received in transfusion. As one respondent put it, autologous donation is "good risk management." Some respondents, particularly the regular blood donors, also mentioned that autologous donation was a way to avoid the depletion of the blood supply, which they regarded as needed primarily for emergencies.

Like anonymous donation and the transfusion of allogenic blood, autologous blood involves certain, albeit different, risks. Patients who use autologous donation are more likely to receive a transfusion than others undergoing the same procedure, because they are more likely to have low hemoglobin levels as a result of the earlier blood donations (Graham et al. 1999; Forgie et al. 1998). In other words, the act of pre-depositing blood creates depletion and a need for that same blood. Treloar and colleagues (2001) identified a tendency for patients to receive their blood back even when there were no strong clinical indications that it was needed, a tendency that arises perhaps from a sense that the blood "belongs" to and should be returned to the patient. So while autologous patients are sequestered from transfusion-related HIV and hepatitis C infection, they are nevertheless more likely to be exposed to the general risks associated with blood transfusion, including the risk of inadvertent mismatch and bacterial infection during surgery (Graham et al. 1999).

We can see here the creation of a new, distinctive variation on the theme of the gift: the gift of self to self. The allogenic blood economy locates a tissue surplus in the bodies of others, who have a collective capacity to regenerate blood and so can afford to give a small amount to the blood bank. The autologous blood economy locates a tissue surplus in the body's capacity to regenerate its own blood over time, and so accumulate enough blood for surgery. The autologous blood economy *withdraws* the donor-recipient from the allogeneic gift economy articulated by Titmuss. It represents the convergence of tissue banking and financial banking: with autologous donation, the bank does not engage in a redistributive role but acts as the manager of an individual deposit-and-withdrawal system. The autologous form of tissue banking has also developed in other tissue economies. We discuss this at greater length in chapter 4.

In contrast to the ethics of generosity and trust advocated for so long by the blood services, the Department of Health in Britain has recently recast autologous donation as an act of civic responsibility and good clinical practice. Autologous donation, its advocates say, not only protects the donor from exposure to the risk of infection but also protects the allogenic blood supply from nonemergency use. Current guidelines for blood management issued by the Department of Health focus on "the use of effective alternatives to donor blood" (United Kingdom, Department of Health 2002, 2). They support the expansion of autologous services as a way to "avoid unnecessary use of donor blood in clinical practice," and to generally conserve blood in the context of the as yet unknown threat that vCJD poses to the blood supply (United Kingdom, Department of Health 2002, 5).

The growing autologous blood economy is highly expressive of a shift in the relationship between blood banks and citizens, one precipitated by the legitimation crisis of blood and its institutions. One the one hand, blood banks have had to fully analyze and acknowledge their responsibilities as complex technical systems, in which changing biotechnologies of blood management have material consequences for the kinds of social relations and forms of health and illness produced. Developments in blood technology and business regimes during the 1970s and 1980s positioned blood banks at the intersection of new global, intercorporeal flows. Blood safety could no longer be guaranteed by social trust between citizens in a defined national space, but rather was hostage to intricate and mutable forms of circulation and transformation throughout the globe, forms of circulation that necessarily produce risk because of their inherent incalculability (Beck 1992). In the wake of this change and its tragic consequences, blood banks have had to pay compensation to the transfusion recipients who contracted AIDS, and transform themselves into highly geared riskmanagement institutions.

On the other hand, the obligations and demands that blood banks place upon their constituencies have become far more prudential. For Titmuss, the gift economy of blood could only function through the uncalculating generosity of the donor, and that donor's understanding of himself or herself within a network of blood redistribution constituted as relations between fellow citizens. Under present conditions, the obligations placed on donors and recipients fall into line with the prudential, risk-averse ethics that Rose and Novas (2004) ascribe to contemporary forms of "biological citizenship." They define biological citizenship as "those citizenship projects that have linked their conceptions of citizens to beliefs about the biological existence of human beings, as individuals, as families and lineages, as communities, as population" (Rose and Novas 2004, 440). The citizenship associated with contemporary blood donation demands that both donors and recipients be fully cognizant of their position, not only within networks of civil obligation but also within networks of risk. Blood donation still calls upon the generosity of donors, but it also obliges donors to both estimate their own risk through screening procedures, and accept that they will find out their risk status because their blood will be tested.

The active endorsement of autologous donation by the blood services in Britain suggests that transfusion recipients too are being encouraged to position themselves with regard to risk, and the value of the blood supply more generally. Allogenic blood has become simultaneously more expensive, because of the costs of screening and testing, and less available, because of dwindling donor pools. Thus allogenic blood has become more valuable, despite being perceived as inherently risky. Autologous blood donation creates a parallel, predictable form of blood collection alongside the allogenic blood supply, so that allogenic blood can be treated as an emergency resource, the last resort when all other blood options are exhausted. Autologous donation both sequesters the patient from the risks of participation in allogenic networks and protects the allogenic blood supply from unnecessary demand. To give to oneself becomes, under these circumstances, an act of prudential, risk-averse citizenship. The generous donor-citizen of *The Gift Relationship* appears, from this vantage point, to be reckless and irresponsible.

2

Disentangling

the Embryonic Gift

THE UK STEM CELL BANK

In chapter 1 we saw that tissue banks could become the site of conflict between different regimes of value. The Alder Hey hospital scandal was provoked by the institution's failure to recognize either the epistemological value of the tissue collection or its ontological significance for bereaved parents. It *underestimated* its collection's significance in both orders of value. The blood contamination scandals of the 1980s were provoked by the various banks' failures to recognize that their existing systems of collection and distribution privileged the rights of donors to give over the rights of recipients to be protected from infection. The blood gift system, understood as inherently ethical and redistributive, involved power relationships that valued the act of donation over the imperatives of public health. Moreover, the banks failed to acknowledge that transnational commodity markets interpenetrated their national gift systems, and that the equation of the gift economy with national identity, safety, and equity was no longer viable.

In this chapter we will discuss a different type of tissue bank recently created in Britain: the UK Stem Cell Bank. The bank's remit is "to curate ethically sourced, quality controlled stem cell lines from all sources on a single site, and make these available to the research community" (Steering Committee of the UK Stem Cell Bank 2004, 10).

Stem cells are types of cell that can renew tissue in the body. Recent biotechnical developments mean that these cells may become sources of transplantable tissue at some point in the future, and the Stem Cell Bank is a major initiative in the British stem cell research effort. Stem cell research is, however, intensely controversial. The most promising stem cells derive from human embryos, and for many people human embryos have a profound ontological significance. While human blood or organs are ethically significant because they *refer to or derive from* a person, many people consider that an embryo *constitutes* a person. Embryos are widely understood as the beginning of human lives.[1] For some people they are already full members of the human community and should be protected from medical research.

Because of this, medical research in Britain and elsewhere involving human embryos takes place in a heavily regulated and sometimes bitterly contested environment. At the same time, embryonic stem cell lines are potential sources of commercial value. Transnational biotechnology companies dominate the research field and trade cell lines around the world. Hence the embryonic stem cell tissue economy is particularly complex and fraught. In this chapter, focused primarily on the British situation, we will examine the vicissitudes of this tissue economy. After describing the technical features of stem cell research, and the broad political context for it in Europe and the United States, we will employ the analytic categories of economic "entanglement" and "disentanglement" posited by Michel Callon (1998) to explore how embryos move from the human body to clinics, laboratory, and stem cell banks. We will then consider the place of the UK Stem Cell Bank in managing its complex regimes of ontological, ethical, therapeutic, and commercial value. We argue that the bank performs a complex double role. On the one hand, it assists in the technical work of disentangling tissues from individuals by facilitating the donation, standardization, and global circulation of stem cells. Yet on the other hand, it performs ethical work that involves a certain reentanglement, for by placing certain limits on the marketing of cell lines and the commercialization of research, it attempts to divert the epistemological value of research into the categories of the public good and the national health. Moreover, it attempts to ameliorate the potential loss of imagined community thrown up for embryo donors by the open-ended nature of stem cell lines, their lack of specifiable spatial or temporal limits.

Embryonic Stem Cell Lines: Biology and Biopolitics The term "stem cell" refers to any cell that can renew tissue in the body. The type most prominent in the media at present is the "pluripotent" stem cell, an undifferentiated cell that has the capacity to develop into almost all of the body's tissue types. Some recent biomedical developments suggest that it may be possible to produce large numbers of undifferentiated stem cells that differentiate on demand, providing an unlimited supply of transplantable tissue. Medical researchers think that stem cells may be very useful in treating currently intransigent medical conditions—Parkinson's disease, Alzheimer's disease, stroke, spinal cord injuries, arthritis—through the introduction of tissue into damaged sites. Stem cells might provide alternative therapies for common conditions like diabetes, promoting the growth of insulin-producing tissue to replace pharmaceutical regimes. They may act as substitutes for organ donation, so that an existing heart or kidney can be repaired rather than replaced. Moreover, it may be possible to produce stem cell lines that are genetically and immunologically compatible with particular hosts, thus avoiding the problem of tissue typing found in organ transplants (McLaren 2000; Vogel 2004).

As we have already noted, the most viable source of stem cell lines is human embryos. Stem cells are found in blood from the umbilical cord and from some adult tissues such as bone marrow, but these other sources do not appear to be as flexible or active as tissue derived from embryos. In vitro fertilization (IVF) programs, which routinely produce large numbers of in vitro embryos, are the major source of embryonic tissue for stem cell research around the world. IVF routinely produces more embryos than can be used in actual reproduction, and in the United Kingdom couples who have completed IVF treatment can donate these "spare" embryos for research. Embryos at this early stage of development are composed exclusively of pluripotent stem cells.

Embryos donated for stem cell research are not kept intact, but disaggregated into individual stem cells. These cells are then immortalized. Immortalization is a technique for growing living tissue in a laboratory.[2] Immortalized cells divide and multiply in vitro, without forming organized tissues like organs or veins. Cells converted into an immortalized cell line will, in theory, divide and multiply forever. Embryonic stem cell lines are immortalized at the point prior to tissue differentiation, while they are still pluripotent. In the experiment that established the first human embryonic stem cell lines (Thomson et al. 1998), cells were cultured for five months without differentiation, then induced to differentiate into the main groups of embryonic tissue layers. Subsequent experiments have induced stem cell lines to differentiate into the precursors of several mature tissue types, including neurons (Reubinoff et al. 2001; Schulz et al. 2003). So immortalization permits the arrest and immobilization of undifferentiated stem cells and the reactivation of differentiating activity on command. It also expands stem cell biomass to usable levels, so that the single "spare" embryo, with two hundred cells, forms the starting point for a significant amount of tissue. A single cell line can be subdivided indefinitely and used to create other lines in other laboratories.

These qualities make stem cell lines very promising therapeutic agents. However, as we have already noted, stem cell research is globally controversial. Stem cell technologies have inherited many of the controversies that have historically circulated around the fetus in abortion debates, regarding the status of the *conceptus* in the human community. Debates in the United Kingdom and elsewhere have focused on whether an embryo has claims to human status, and the kinds of legal and ethical protections that it deserves. The public and commentators have expressed anxieties about biotechnical intervention in the beginnings of human life, and the instrumentalization of embryos—their use for medical ends that do not serve their own interests (Habermas 2003; Mulkay 1997). As patentable entities, stem cell lines have also inherited a set of controversies regarding the commercialization of human reproductive material, interpreted as the commodification of human life (Knowles and Adams 2001–2).

Stem cell technologies are also contaminated by their association with the new cloning technologies made famous by the birth of Dolly the sheep. Dolly was cloned through a process called cell nuclear replacement, which creates an embryo not by the usual process of conception—the fusion of egg and sperm—but by inserting the nucleus of a cell from adult tissue into an oocyte, or unfertilized egg. This process creates an embryo with the genetic profile of the donor adult. In Dolly's case, in a practice termed reproductive cloning, the embryo was introduced into the uterus of a surrogate mother, who carried it to term, producing a genetic copy of the gene donor. It may be possible to use some aspects of this technique to develop embryonic stem cell lines with the genetic material of an adult donor. Such a practice, known as therapeutic cloning, would produce transplantable tissues genetically compatible with the donor, and so avoid the problem of immunological rejection that plagues all forms of tissue transplant. Advocates of stem cell technologies make careful distinctions between therapeutic cloning for producing stem cells and reproductive cloning for producing whole new creatures. Nevertheless, the distinctions are highly volatile and the term "cloning" has attracted a general public opprobrium that is largely indifferent to such distinctions.[3]

Despite these controversies, most of the advanced industrial democracies have developed some kind of regulatory framework to facilitate stem cell research. The medical and political interest in stem cell technologies arises from their promise to address two difficult biopolitical problems. The first problem is the increasing difficulty of mobilizing organ donations in the face of ever-growing demand. While rates of organ donation have increased slightly in many developed countries over the last ten years, the demand for organs has far outstripped supply (World Health Organization 2003). In addition to the recurrent problems of tissue typing and transporting highly perishable organs to locations where they are needed, waiting lists lengthen because of what Renée Fox describes as the "aspiration to transplant . . . to replace every worn out part of the human body" (quoted in Stafford 1999, 243–44). Stem cell tissue promises to ameliorate these problems because, in theory at least, it is a self-renewing and flexible substance. As one article puts it, stem cells could act as "universal donor cells . . . 'off the shelf' reagent, prepared and/or additionally engineered under good manufacturing practices readily available in limitless quantities for the acute phases of an injury or disease" (Snyder and Vescovi 2000, 828). Stem cells are imagined as an unlimited resource, the precise opposite of singular organs.

The second biopolitical problem is the aging of populations in developed nations. By 2020 approximately 20 percent of the population in the G8 nations will be over sixty-five (Neilson 2003), and they will live longer than previous generations. As Neilson points out, this shift in the demographic profile of the industrial democracies presents a set of intractable policy problems to governments: "With portentous consequences for the ratio of working-age taxpayers to nonworking retirees, these changes in age profile threaten the economic viability of the world's wealthiest and most powerful nation-states, tearing at the fabric of their once liberal notions of citizenship, constitutionalism, and social contracturalism. . . . population aging places a glacier-like pressure on the nation-state, slowly but surely eroding its centralized apparatuses for managing the production and reproduction of life" (Neilson 2003, 163).

Aging populations place large burdens on the provision of welfare and pensions. At the same time, many governments have reduced immigration (though it has the potential to enlarge the tax base and increase reproduction rates), in response to fears about social disorder and global terrorism. Aging populations also present specific health problems. More and more people develop chronic and degenerative conditions associated with aging—stroke, Parkinson's disease, Alzheimer's disease, and heart disease. Health systems devote an increasing proportion of their budgets to the long-term management of such conditions (Chief Medical Officer's Expert Group 2000), as people live longer with more disease. These are precisely the kinds of conditions that stem cell technology, and the field of regenerative medicine more generally, promise to treat. Stem cell technologies, as Sperling (2004) and Cooper (2006) point out, carry with them an aura of potential, both at the microbiological level (the potential to endlessly proliferate and differentiate) and the macro-social level (as governments have seized on their potential to regenerate the vitality of aging populations).

As a consequence, most of the industrial democracies have regulatory regimes and some degree of public funding to facilitate stem cell research. Configurations of funding and regulation vary widely. In the United States pressure from right-to-life groups and a historical absence of moral consensus about the status of embryos and fetuses have placed severe restrictions on federal funding for stem cell research (Gottweis 2002). In August 2001 President Bush declared that federal funding for stem cell research would be made available only for the approximately sixty sets of stem cell lines extant at the time, for which "life and death decisions have already been made" (Bush 2001). This constitutes a significant restriction, as many of these lines are not considered viable for research (Agres 2003). In contrast, embryonic stem cell research is largely unregulated in the private sector in the United States, and as a result significant research is primarily located or funded there (Gottweis 2002). Recently, state legislatures in the United States have circumvented the federal restrictions by providing public funds for stem cell research, often to public-private research partnerships (Hogle 2004).

Throughout the member states of the European Union, national policies range from prohibiting all embryonic stem cell research (Ireland, Spain, France), to providing public funds under strict limitations (Austria, Denmark), to funding therapeutic cloning research (United Kingdom) (Salter and Jones 2002). In Germany a particularly difficult debate about embryonic stem cell research has been couched in anxieties about eugenics, "Nazi medicine," the social acceptance of disabled people, and the human rights of the embryo. Organized opposition to embryonic stem cell research comes from the churches, several political parties of both left and right, and the German president. In 2002 the Bundestag voted to support the importation of embryonic stem cell lines from other nations for research under very strict limits, a decision that remains controversial (Gottweis 2002). Recently the EU Framework 6 funding program has made public funds available for embryonic stem cell research, although it will not support the creation of embryos for research purposes.

These systems of public, national funding for embryonic stem cell research sit alongside significant transnational, commercial investments. Embryonic stem cell lines are patentable in the United Kingdom, the United States, and a number of other advanced industrial nations; companies like ES Cell International, based in Singapore, and Advanced Cell Technology and Geron, based in the United States, currently hold the licenses to patents on the majority of existing stem cell lines. To date more than five hundred patent applications for human embryonic stem cell lines have been filed worldwide (Caulfield

2003). In most cases, public funding for stem cell research is designed to work together with commercial research rather than to replace it, and public sector researchers also secure patents on their stem cell lines.

Stem Cell Research in the United Kingdom   The United Kingdom is at the forefront of the public sector research program, in part because of a history of public debate and sometimes tenuous social consensus around the use of embryonic tissues for medical research. Since the publication in 1984 of the Warnock Report on the legal and ethical aspects of assisted human reproduction, there has been vigorous debate around research on embryos, a debate that resulted in the Human Fertilisation and Embryology Act of 1990 and the establishment of the Human Fertilisation and Embryology Authority (HFEA) to administer it. The act established a regulatory framework for the practice of in vitro fertilization and the management of IVF embryos, including the use of supernumerary embryos for research into reproductive health. Researchers may only use embryos for the first fourteen days after conception, or until the development of the primitive streak, the beginnings of a neurological system. Research laboratories must be licensed by the HFEA, and contravention of the act may incur criminal sanctions (Mulkay 1997). This use of the criminal code is in keeping with the "special status of the embryo" and "the respect which is due to human life at all stages of its development" (Human Fertilisation and Embryology Authority 2001, 7). In this respect, the HFEA oversees a regulatory regime that recognizes the epistemological and ontological regimes of value underlying the research embryo's significance, and tries to configure them in non-oppositional ways. Like the definition of brain death that allows the harvesting of viable organs from donor cadavers, the fourteen-day limit provides a margin of usable vitality, a pragmatic boundary between nonhuman and proto-human status.

With the creation of the first human embryonic stem cell lines in 1998, the potential applications of embryo research multiplied dramatically, and after further public debate the HFEA was extended, in 2001, to allow for stem cell research. Under the expanded act, supernumerary embryos may be used for research into serious disease (primarily interpreted as degenerative conditions like Alzheimer's and Parkinson's disease) and the development of treatments. The act allows both therapeutic cloning and the creation of embryos for research purposes, under specific conditions. Consequently, the United Kingdom now has the most liberal regime for stem cell research among countries that regulate biotechnology.

This success in keeping embryo research within acceptable social limits and under well-managed governance has given the United Kingdom a strong position in the international research arena. The creation of the Stem Cell Bank is seen as an important part of an overall strategy to consolidate this position.[4] All laboratories licensed for stem cell research must deposit viable cell lines with the bank. It will work at both a national and an international level, making stem cell lines available to researchers worldwide, and recruiting international researchers to deposit their lines in the bank. It remains to be seen whether international depositors will use the bank, but researchers in Australia, Canada, and other nations have indicated an interest in doing so.[5]

The bank has a complex technical brief: to assess the viability of lines, assess the complex medical risks associated with therapeutic tissues, maintain a master bank of cells, and distribute the cells throughout the world. It also has a complex ethical brief. The bank must oversee the ethical derivation of the embryos and cell lines, including international lines, and ensure that researchers use stem cell lines for appropriate, nontrivial forms of research. It must ensure that lines are not derived unnecessarily, and that the minimum number of embryos is used to create the optimum number of cell lines. To put it in terms we have already developed, the bank must manage both the technicity of stem cell lines and the complex politics of value that they involve.

Tissue Banking: Entangled and Disentangled Tissues   Michel Callon, in his study of the technologies of markets (Callon 1998),[6] has described the economies of human organ transplantation as "entangled." Organs cannot be stored outside the body for any length of time, and the way they move between donor and recipient must be very direct and inflexible. The organ must be removed from the (usually brain-dead) donor as quickly as possible, rushed to the recipient, and transplanted immediately. In this sense organs present the most restricted kind of tissue economy—one person gives to another, through anonymous hospital protocols, in real time, with as little change to the organ as possible. Callon suggests that we think of this economy as "entangled," for the movement of organs is severely restricted by their immunological particularity, as well as their nonstandard, perishable nature and their profound involvement in kinship, mortality, affect, and bodily relations. He describes this very restricted circulation as the symmetrical opposite of currency circulation, which works to "disentangle." Money, as pure exchange value without use value of its own, circulates anonymously, changing from hand to hand, indefinitely substitutable for itself. Money, Callon argues, serves to disentangle objects from their owners by providing equivalence. It facilitates market forms of circulation in which buyers and sellers strike a price, complete their transaction, and are quits—they do not remain in relationship once they complete the transaction. The commodity may continue in some form of circulation, moving from buyer to seller through the mechanism of money. Solid organs, by contrast, circulate in the most personal and time-limited form. Callon asks, "how is it possible to circulate a liver, a kidney or a heart, between a donor—generally dead—and a recipient—generally in danger of death—when the organ is entangled in the body of a potential donor and through him in his family or circle of friends? The transfer of the organ is a forcing out in the true sense of the term; its success depends on that of disentanglement. The difficulty of this disentanglement explains why the transfer is most often in the form of a gift, which . . . reconciles circulation and entanglement" (Callon 1998, 36).

For Callon, the donation of such entangled organs is a means of putting them into play, initiating a limited form of circulation that honors the material and social embeddedness of organs.[7] However, he argues, no entity can exist in a state of perfect disentanglement or entanglement. Money both constitutes relations through loans and gifts, and leaves a paper trail of its trajectory that is itself a map of social transactions. Organs, particularly kidneys, can be constituted as commodities, bought and sold on sometimes illicit global markets (Scheper-Hughes 2000; Scheper-Hughes 2002b). Callon's framework is useful because it suggests some ways to think about the different implications of bankable and nonbankable tissue circulation. Tissue banks can be thought of as technical institutions that assist in the work of partially disentangling human tissues from the network of embodied social relations in which they originate, and freeing them up to circulate through the body politic in more complex and flexible ways than is possible for whole organs.

Disentangling the Embryo: Donation, Informed Consent, and Proto-commodities   Embryos are, like organs, entangled entities, emerging out of embodied social relations. However, unlike solid organs they are also open to technical and legal forms of disentanglement. They can be transformed into a stem cell line that can be banked, copied, and circulated, and constituted as the intellectual property of the researcher. This latter form of disentanglement also involves a profound transmutation in value, as the ontological significance of the embryo and the social value of its donation give way to the investment value of the patented cell line. Patent protects research innovation, but it also confers on cell lines and other biological entities an aura of potential value that makes them negotiable assets for both public and commercial research laboratories. Thus embryos can be disentangled into stem cell lines according to market logics.

In its mode of production, the IVF embryo is profoundly entangled. Couples undertake IVF in the context of the sense of loss, inadequacy, and grief attendant on the realization of infertility (Throsby 2004). In Britain public funding through the National Health Service is somewhat patchy, and couples often pay for cycles of IVF themselves. The couple, and particularly the woman, produces the embryo through intense and demanding emotional and bodily labor. IVF involves lengthy, often grueling procedures—complex drug regimes to suppress pituitary function, stimulate the follicles, and cause hyperovulation, numerous appointments at the clinic, extended time away from work, egg harvesting, and implantation. The couple endures these procedures in a cycle of hope and despair, and even repeated use of IVF has only an 18 percent chance of producing a child (Throsby 2002a; Throsby 2002b; Throsby 2004). In this respect the IVF embryo signifies a hoped-for child, and is enmeshed in an intensely particular web of affect, kinship relations, and embodiment. However, the embryo is also an in vitro entity, conceived in a petri dish and, if not implanted immediately, stored in a freezer. Thus it also exists as a biotechnical entity in a web of laboratory relations. It could be transformed into a cell line and circulated through the global technical networks of biomedical research, but only if it is disentangled from the personal relations that produced it, and from its significance as a potentially implantable entity, a possible future child.

This first step in the process of disentanglement therefore depends on the couple's decision to transfer "spare" embryos to a research program. Couples must give rather than sell their embryos because, as we have discussed, in Britain giving tissues is understood as better social policy than selling tissues, a fundamental act of citizenship and community. This understanding of the social value generated by *giving* tissues is frequently restated in policy documents and guidelines around human tissue management. For example, the current *Operational and Ethical Guidelines on the Use of Human Tissues for Research* of the Medical Research Council state, "We recommend that tissue samples donated for research be treated as gifts or donations, although gifts with conditions attached. This is preferable from a moral and ethical point of view as it promotes the 'gift relationship' between research participants and scientists, and underlies the altruistic motivation for participation in research" (Medical Research Council 2001, 8).

Here the guidelines restate Titmuss's argument, while at the same time glossing over a very significant difference. This is not a gift of life to a fellow citizen, but a gift of potential knowledge to a medical researcher. Laurie (2001), in his legal overview of recent inquiries into tissue retention and research in Britain,[8] notes that each report adopts the gift-with-consent model for the transfer of human tissues from the person to the researcher, and that this system is universally preferred over a property model. Moreover, in English common law persons do not have property rights in their own bodies, and cannot sell a part of themselves. The human body and its parts are considered beyond commerce and outside of contract, and once tissue has left the body, it is understood to belong to no one (Dickenson 2002; Lawrence 1998). This principle is further enshrined in civil legislation like the Human Tissue Act of 2004, which prohibits the sale of organs and tissues for transplant.

Thus anyone who wishes to transfer tissues to another party must do so as a gift.[9] However, as we have already seen, human tissues are more and more likely to be engineered in complex ways by medical researchers, not directly reincorporated into another person. Tissue donors may find that their donation goes neither directly to another person, as with whole organ donation, nor indirectly to another person, via a tissue bank. Instead it goes to a laboratory that biotechnically transforms the material. In the case of embryo donation for stem cell research, the embryo is simply the starting point for an expandable network of cell lines whose destination is unknowable.

It is at this point, the gift of tissues to research laboratories, when issues of property come to the fore. While persons have no property rights in their own body parts, it is possible for a second party to establish property rights in tissues once they have left the donor's body. The House of Lords Select Committee Report on Stem Cell Research cites *Regina v. Kelly* (1998) to support this proposition, while not overturning the common law principle that a person may only establish property rights in another person's removed body parts by transforming the material through a process of skill.[10]

Informed consent is the mechanism that transforms a gift into property. This initially may seem counterintuitive, for informed consent is also the central bioethical principle governing a patient's relationship to participation in biomedical research, "the principal code to be adhered to so as to protect the individual patient or healthy volunteer subject from possible exploitation and harm" (Corrigan 2003). Under the principle of informed consent, a person has the right to be fully informed about the possible dangers and risks of participation in medical research, and the opportunity to give or refuse consent. The principle of informed consent is understood to protect the autonomy and dignity of the individual, and to prevent coercion, medical paternalism, and exploitation (Lupton 1997; Corrigan 2003). Thus when donors give tissues for research, the informed consent procedure is explicitly designed to protect them from exploitative medical pressure.

However, we contend that the procedure also performs a quite different function, allied to the commercial aspects of tissue research. *It serves to regulate and formalize the transfer of possession from donor to recipient.* The *Operational and Ethical Guidelines on the Use of Human*

Tissues for Research state this function of donation quite frankly: "We recommend that tissue samples donated for research be treated as gifts or donations . . . [This] provides a practical way of dealing with the legal uncertainty over ownership, in that any property rights that the donor might have in their donated sample would be transferred, together with the control of use of the sample, to the recipient of the gift. . . . It is very important that the donor understands and agrees to the proposed uses of the donated material" (Medical Research Council 2001, 8). Under the guidelines, the informed consent procedure combines protection of the donor with the transfer of legal claim to the tissue. While donors may freely give tissues, they forfeit all further claims to them in the act of donation. The gift is not reversible and cannot be reclaimed, nor can the giver claim residual rights in what has been given. The gift, once given, ceases to refer to the donor. Here the informed consent procedure acts as a kind of surrogate property contract.

With regard to embryos donated for stem cell research, the standard Donor Information and Consent Form clearly states that once the embryo has been donated, the donor has no further claims on it. In particular, the donor relinquishes any rights to future commercial value of embryonic products: "You will receive no financial reward from future commercial application of such research. . . . In the future, stem cell lines derived from donated embryos might be used to develop new treatments, including cell replacement therapy. It will not be possible to turn this research into new treatments that will provide widespread health benefits without involving commercial companies. Cell lines and developments arising from stem cell research might be patented by academic researchers or commercial companies. However, the research and development process involves many stages and the contribution of your individual embryo(s) to any future profits will be impossible to quantify."[11] Moreover, in the case of embryonic stem cells the logic of informed consent dovetails with the requirements for establishing intellectual property rights through the patenting of biological entities. As we discuss at greater length in chapter 3, since the U.S. Supreme Court ruling in *Diamond v. Chakrabarty* (1980), it has been possible to patent biotechnically engineered tissues and entities if they fulfill the criteria for invention—they must be novel, useful, and non-obvious. Entities as diverse as gene sequences, single nucleotide polymorphisms, cell lines, and multicellular organisms like knockout mice have been patented under these criteria. Biotechnology patents may generate considerable investment funds and profits for their holders, while at the same time the donors themselves cannot make claims on the productivity of their material.

Embryonic stem cell lines are patentable entities in the United Kingdom. The patent office has ruled that the embryo is not itself patentable, nor are totipotent[12] embryonic cells that could still give rise to an embryo. However pluripotent cells can form the basis for a patentable cell line, on the grounds that "they do not have the potential to develop into an entire human body" and thus "the commercial exploitation of inventions concerning human embryonic pluripotent stem cells would not be contrary to public policy or morality in the United Kingdom."[13]

In summary, while legal and bioethical debate continues around whether informed consent better protects donors' rights than a system based on property rights (Laurie 2001) in our analysis, *informed consent is already based on property rights: the rights of the recipient*. This is the crucial distinction noted earlier between the gift in Titmuss's sense—the gift to a fellow citizen—and the gift to medical researchers—the gift as a covert form of property, to which only the receiving party can lay claim. However, this inequitable contractual aspect of the informed consent process is largely suppressed.

Intellectual Property and the Repression of the Gift   Informed consent thus dissociates the embryo from the network of family relations that produced it, and positions it as a technical entity whose productivity is at the disposal of the laboratory. The next step in the process of disentanglement is its transformation into a cell line. As a cell line, it can be standardized, stored, divided, multiplied, and transported throughout the world. It may eventually be reincorporated as a therapy into numerous bodies. This transformation is also the "inventive step" that distinguishes the cell line from a mere discovery and qualifies it for patent. The establishment of intellectual property rights is crucial if biomedical researchers are to entice venture capital into their laboratories, capital considered essential to develop basic, public sector research into deliverable therapies. As noted in the guidelines of the Medical Research Council (the major source of public funds for biomedical research in Britain), "The MRC's mission is to support research that will ultimately benefit human health. The development of new drug therapies, and diagnostic and screening tests, to the point where they can be made sufficiently widely available to benefit human health, is crucially dependant on commercial involvement" (Medical Research Council 2001, 12).

Patent provides a way for laboratories to protect their inventive work from competitors and for investors to profit from the commercialization of research. It also involves a further process of disentanglement in favor of the research laboratory and the market, by means of which the contribution of the donors, and of the embryonic material itself, is dissociated from the productivity of the stem cell line. Intellectual property in biological entities is organized through a mind-body split that makes the contribution of the body—in the case of embryo donation, primarily the woman's body—understood as dumb matter that must be animated by the contribution of mind. As Strathern (1999) observes, the concept of intellectual property, particularly in living material, depends on separating the ideational content from the material that it is said to transform: "The significance of the added element that turns 'nature's handiwork' into the inventor's has its antecedents in an ancient cosmology of animation: matter requires form. Form appears as ideational, as potential, precisely when it is not matter or materialization" (Strathern 1999, 176).

The House of Lords Select Committee Report on Stem Cell Research, the report that founded the Stem Cell Bank, gives unequivocal endorsement to this understanding: "It has been suggested that those who donate an embryo for stem cell research might subsequently expect a share in any benefits accruing from commercial exploitation of research on stem cell lines derived from it. In our view, it would be undesirable for legislation to permit such claims: any commercial benefits will have come about as a result of the research and subsequent development rather than any intrinsic quality of a particular embryo donated. However, it makes it even more important that potential donors should fully understand the implications if embryos they are donating may be used for the production of stem cell lines" (House of Lords 2002, paragraph 8.32).

The contribution made by the donated material itself, and the donor's work in producing that material, is systematically devalued in this way of organizing the distinction between discovery and invention. We have already described the process of producing a "spare" embryo, the emotional, financial, and physical labor performed by the donors, especially the woman. This production also requires highly specialized technical labor, and the resources of a clinic and a laboratory. Nevertheless, in the organization of intellectual property this work is devalued, because it only produces the "natural" object, the embryo. Furthermore, the value of the embryonic material, and its particular kind of self-organizing and differentiating properties, are repressed in this organization of patent. As Habermas puts it, biotechnology involves *collaboration* between the capacities of living matter and technology, not the technical replacement or animation of living matter (Habermas 2003). Embryonic stem cell lines have therapeutic potential because of the specifically pluripotent nature of the tissues cultured, a quality not found in other kinds of more dedicated tissues. The embryonic stem cell line is productive because it transposes this potential and reorganizes its conditions of reproduction. Pottage (1998) makes a similar point with regard to the PNG-1 patent, the now notorious attempt to patent a T-cell line derived from the blood of a Papua New Guinean tribesman:[14] "Given that the innovative content of this invention seems to owe more to the natural components of the extracted materials than to any technological process of extraction and purification, the idea that the production of the cell line involved a radically inventive process seems particularly implausible. Unlike the more complex and precarious achievements of recombinant DNA technology, the production of an immortal cell line demands little more of the inventor than the mastery of a routine scientific technique. The 'inventive' process seems merely to transcribe a natural code into a new medium" (Pottage 1998, 752).

Patented embryonic stem cell lines are thus established through a mind-body split and a systematic denial of indebtedness to the embryo donors or to the productivity of the embryonic material itself. Both this split and this denial assume the biology and provenance of the gift without acknowledging it. Moreover, it is precisely the split and the denial that serve as the differential powering the engine of contemporary commercial tissue economies. Under these conditions of donation and patent, tissue donors are effectively open sources of biological material, which can be readily disentangled in ways that favor the rights and profits of biotechnology companies.

The Stem Cell Bank: Re-entangling Stem Cell Lines The Stem Cell Bank intervenes in these complicated processes of disentanglement in two seemingly opposed ways. On the one hand, it is a key institution in the process of disentangling the embryo from its particular social context. After the donation and the consent and laboratory processes are completed, the bank is the site where the cell lines will be anonymized, characterized, and standardized. It will propel cell lines into national and transnational circulation, generating working cell lines from master cell banks. It will act as a neutral intermediary between depositing and withdrawing parties with regard to intellectual property arrangements. The bank's Code of Practice states: "the UK Stem Cell Bank will not take any direct interest in intellectual property embodied in deposited cell lines, or become involved in the negotiations between depositors and users" (Steering Committee of the UK Stem Cell Bank 2004, 38). In this sense, the bank will facilitate intellectual property agreements, but will not intervene in them.

On the other hand, the bank also facilitates the reentanglement of stem cells by tying them to imagined communities. It will harness stem cell research in the United Kingdom to purposes of national health, and oversee the ethical management of stem cell lines in ways that recognize their ontological and familial origins. To put it another way, the bank will solicit potential donors to give their embryos, precisely by reentangling embryonic stem cell lines in webs of social obligation and imagined community. As we have seen, many technical, commercial, and legal features of the stem cell economy constitute obstacles to embryo donation, precisely because they appear to dissociate the embryo from the values of generosity, kinship, and human community associated with the act of embryo production and donation.

In particular, we argue, the technicity of stem cell lines makes it difficult for donors to imagine the beneficiaries of their gift. Who is the recipient of the donation? To use Titmuss's elegant formulation, "Who is my stranger?" What is the relationship between donor and recipients in stem cell research? Donors who give their embryos for reproductive medical research instead of stem cell research can readily identify, and identify *with*, the final beneficiaries of their gift: other couples involved in fertility treatment. The immediate material recipient of the embryo, the clinic and laboratory, is a stable site for the benefit of the infertile. Donors could also place conditions on their donation, specifying it for a particular program of research. Thus the embryonic gift to reproductive medical research has a relatively stable destination, a set of uses, and a specifiable group of beneficiaries. It is a gift circulating in a limited way within a viable imagined community of infertility medicine and infertile couples, a form of circulation readily reconciled with its entangled status.

With stem cell research, however, any given line may be dispersed to multiple researchers around the world. They may maintain the line for an unspecifiable period, and use it for research in areas as diverse as spinal injury, diabetes, organ regeneration, or Parkinson's disease. Each cell line perpetuates the donor couple's joint genetic material, and as an immortalized line, this genetic material can remain viable long after both members of the donor couple die. It is immortalized but they are not. So a donated embryo may be the starting point for an unknowable, infinitely branching network of cell lines, propagating the donors' DNA, with no specific destination and no time horizon. Uses may be found for cell lines that are impossible to anticipate under current technical conditions. For this reason, donors to stem cell research programs will not be able to select which projects use their embryos.

Recent research among potential embryo donors confirms the difficulties presented by this set of features (People Science and Policy 2003).[15] Women and men who had experienced IVF stated their willingness to donate spare embryos for reproductive medical research, as a way to help others in the same situation and to repay the benefits they had received from previous research. The participants were less willing to donate to open-ended research: the implications of immortalization disturbed them, particularly the impossibility of consenting in the present to research in the distant future. They were anxious that cell lines might be used for trivial or commercially driven research, or for unacceptable practices like reproductive cloning.

It seems to us that the UK Stem Cell Bank presents one part of a solution to the problems of governance, commercial exploitation, and imagined community created by the unbounded, disentangled nature of the embryonic stem cell economy. It does this in a number of ways. First, as we described earlier, it will play an important role in ethical oversight of the stem cell economy. The bank's Steering Committee will evaluate the informed consent procedures and other patient protection protocols tendered with each deposited cell line, to ensure they comply with HFEA requirements for protecting both donor and embryo. In addition, the bank will ensure that stem cell lines are not created needlessly. The problem of tissue matching means that a wide genetic array of stem cell material may be needed to match any one patient, as many as four thousand according to some estimates (Vogel 2002, 1784). This means that researchers will need access to a spectrum of cell lines. One of the major functions of the bank will be to offer a library of available cell lines to researchers, maximizing their access to different lines and preempting any need for individual laboratories to produce diversity in-house. The House of Lords Select Committee Report on Stem Cell Research (2002) identifies one of the major advantages of a stem cell bank as its ability to "minimize the need to generate new [embryonic stem] cell lines (and consequently minimize the use of embryos for research) while not impeding scientific and medical progress" (paragraph 8.24). The embryo donor consent form stresses this aspect of the bank's function: "Keeping cell lines in a stem cell bank that can be accessed by many scientists will help to reduce the number of embryos that are needed for research. The stem cell lines will be characterized, standardized, frozen and stored for future use in approved research projects, perhaps many years later. . . . All scientists who want to use banked stem cell lines derived from embryos will have to seek approval from a high level Stem Cell Steering Committee. . . . approval will only be given if i) the research is necessary and of high quality, ii) the scientists are following UK legal and ethical guidelines, and iii) the scientists provide evidence that they have secured all essential licences or accreditations from relevant UK ethical and regulatory authorities."[16]

This role is one of the bank's major contributions to managing the stem cell economy. It demonstrates to donors that excessive demand for embryos will be curbed, and the ontological and epistemological significance of each embryonic gift will be highly valued. No embryo will be sacrificed for trivial reasons. No embryonic cell line will be accepted that has not passed through the appropriate informed consent procedures. None will be squandered or used for inappropriate or frivolous ends. Each line will be deployed to maximize its therapeutic usefulness. Participants in focus groups endorsed these functions of the bank, stating that its greatest benefit would be the ethical oversight that it would provide to the uses of the cell lines (People Science and Policy 2003).

The bank should also militate against some of the problems of imagined community presented by the dispersed nature of the stem cell economy. The bank cannot provide an absolute sense of destination, nor can it be the final recipient of the embryonic gift. However, it will provide a stable location for the master cell banks that will generate working cell lines, and a public site where the various possible uses of the tissue will be adjudicated according to principles of public interest and donor protection. In the words of the Medical Research Council guidelines for managing human tissues, the bank can be the custodian of donated material: "If samples taken for research are to be treated as gifts, there must be a recipient, to whom formal responsibility for custodianship . . . is transferred. While the principal investigator should have day-to-day responsibility for management of a collection of human material, the M RC considers that it is more appropriate for formal responsibility for custodianship. . . . to rest with institutions . . . This provides greater security for valuable collections, [and] provides better assurance that donor's rights will be protected" (Medical Research Council 2001, 8).

This custodial model of tissue banking, we argue, helps to stabilize and specify a relationship between embryo donor and potential therapeutic recipients. The bank should also help to secure global research benefits in the interests of British citizens so as not to see them diverted to transnational health markets, as might be done under strictly commercial research. Unlike the blood banks in the 1980s, which continued to act as if their field of operations was strictly national, the UK Stem Cell Bank is set up as an exogenous, global actor, positioned to marshal global flows of stem cell tissues, knowledge, and expertise for national benefit. In this respect the bank will reassure donors that while the cell lines created from their embryonic gift may be distributed throughout the world, the knowledge and therapies generated will be available to fellow citizens.

The bank also sets out management principles that will divert into public sector research institutions what might otherwise be strictly market forms of stem cell circulation. Stem cell lines will be sequestered from market pricing to some extent, and all depositors of cell lines must agree to certain conditions of distribution.[17] These include:

—Cell lines must not be sold for financial gain.
—Depositors are to make lines available to academic researchers with minimal constraints and conditions, and no upfront fees. Fees may be charged for commercial users.
—Public sector researchers will pay the bank the marginal costs of supplying the lines, while commercial users will pay full costs.
—Neither users nor depositors may pass sample lines to third parties without the explicit approval of the Bank steering committee or the HFEA.
—Users of lines must deposit any further cell lines developed with the bank.

These stipulations have several important effects. First, they make the bank a source of low-cost cell lines for public sector researchers, who might otherwise have to purchase lines at the market price. In this way the bank helps to bring stem cell lines within the budget of public sector funding. Second, they should encourage the growth of a research ecology, so that researchers are not deterred from sharing ideas by an overly competitive structure or excessive access costs. The effect should be to facilitate osmosis between public sector researchers, and to lower the barriers between commercial and public sector researchers by giving them access to the same pool of material through a differential pricing structure. As James Boyle (2003) writes, innovation is a collaborative and distributed process. Overly privatized models of research that treat basic research materials as property put up price barriers to access and lower the critical mass of researchers involved in a field. What Boyle terms "high-wall" intellectual property conditions, which place tight restrictions on licensees, also obstruct peer-to-peer engagement and the sharing of research findings. The demand that all researchers deposit any further cell lines developed with the bank is a means of ensuring that innovations made with the assistance of the bank's collection return to a central location, so that other researchers may build on them incrementally. Again, the notion is to contribute to a research ecology, so that researchers gain access to stem cell material and in return contribute their innovations back into a public domain. Third, these conditions ensure that the bank will be an "obligatory passage point" (Latour 1988) through which all embryonic stem cell line circulation in Britain must pass. It gives shape to the potentially infinite proliferation of stem cell lines, and brings all circulation under the purview of the bank's social charter to scrutinize the health objectives of the research. The bank may also become an obligatory passage point for researchers elsewhere in the world, in particular researchers who share the bank's commitment to public oversight of stem cell research.

The embryonic stem cell economy sources tissue from the in vitro embryo, an entity produced at the intersection of kinship relations, reproductive desire, and laboratory technique. At the very margin of earliest human life, the in vitro embryo signifies for many the origin of both the species and the human community, an entity whose proper location is in vivo. For the biosciences and biocommerce, the in vitro embryo signifies potential vitality, self-renewing productivity, an infinite tissue resource, and a locale for investment and profit. Its proper role is to circulate through global research networks as a stem cell line. It is this double life of the in vitro embryo that presents such problems for the social management of its values.

The UK Stem Cell Bank both propels embryonic stem cell lines through global research networks and locates them in a single site and time frame. As the obligatory passage point for all stem cell lines derived in the United Kingdom, the bank can accumulate master cell banks and provide ethical oversight to an entire field of tissue that would otherwise disperse throughout the globe and into an unknowable future. It provides a stable site of governance and brings all the stem cell lines under a single bioethical gaze. As a public institution, the bank will help to locate the stem cell research effort in public, national space, even when commercial firms carry it out. It will try to ensure that British research it is not diverted away from national health boundaries by global markets. To this extent it is well situated to manage, although not resolve, the potential conflicts over embryonic value arising from stem cell circulation. While the bank cannot fundamentally alter the structural inequity built into the giving of tissues to increasingly commercialized research bodies, it may ameliorate and dissipate some of its worst effects. However, the ever-increasing commercial value of the biological fragment presents a serious and complex challenge to all institutions charged with securing human tissue donations. In part II, "Waste and Tissue Economies," we examine two refusals by donors to give their tissues gratuitously. In the first case one person, John Moore, attempted and failed to secure property rights in his spleen tissue. In the second, we explore the lucrative industry that has grown up around parents' desire to secure their children's cord blood as personal property, rather than donate it to public cord-blood banks.

PART II

Waste and

Tissue

Economies

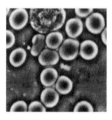 In one of the more striking scenes in David Fincher's film *Fight Club* (1999), the narrator and his partner steal plastic bags of discarded body wastes from a dumpster behind a liposuction clinic. The two convert the fats from this corporeal garbage into soap, which they sell to fashion boutiques for twenty dollars a bar. The narrator positions this commodification of body waste as a subversive maneuver, claiming that "[i]t was beautiful. We were selling rich women their own fat acids [or "fat asses"; the pun is deliberate] back to them." The viewer is no doubt supposed to find this scenario hyperbolic, the satire depending on the notion that we, the viewers, are not yet so gullible that we would pay good money to buy back our own bodily waste after it had been processed through the infrastructure of capitalism and commodity culture.

Yet as our previous chapters have suggested, the tissue economy depicted in this film is no wild imagining of the Hollywood entertainment industry. The recycling and transformation of "waste" tissues—from the sale by hospitals of infant foreskins (used to manufacture artificial skin) and aborted embryo gonads (a source of stem cells) to the patenting of infected cell lines as research materials—is a central dynamic of contemporary tissue economies. This should not be surprising. As several commentators have noted (Hawkins and Mueke 2003; Frow 2003; Thompson 1979), the concept of waste plays a central role in all forms of economy and theories of value. All economies must deal with what appears as waste within their own systems, if they are to remain profitable. "Loss, waste and the unproductive are anti-economic—they disturb the logic of general positivity that defines an economy" (Hawkins and Mueke 2003, xii). Matter classified as rubbish in one domain of an economy, household waste for example, must be transformed into profit in another, through recycling, mulching, landfill, and so on. Waste material which may appear as the very opposite of value in one context can become the starting point for the generation of significant degrees of value in another. Hence one of the fundamental movements of any successful form of economy is the circulation of waste objects from unprofitable to profitable contexts, where they can be resignified and redeployed. Waste, to paraphrase the pronouncement by Douglas (1984) about dirt, "is matter out of place," and the strategic work of any economy involves relocating waste to other regimes of value where it does productive work.

Such a recuperation of waste is evident in many human tissue economies. In chapters 1 and 2 we examined two types of tissue that are emphatically *not* waste—donated blood and embryos. As we saw, these two tissue types are imbued with profound ontological significance—the first designates the altruism and civil status of the donor, the second the beginnings of human life. For this reason, both types are hedged around with complex forms of regulation, and remain largely sequestered from the marketplace at point of donation, although they may subsequently be commodified in various ways. Generally speaking, human tissues are more likely to be classified as waste as they lose ontological significance. Tissues that we consider essential to the body's integrity and function—organs, blood, skin, the limbs—are strongly invested with ontological significance, and their loss is a catastrophe for the subject. Tissues that are routinely shed or expelled by the body—hair and nail clippings, nasal secretions, saliva, pus, skin particles, urine, feces, sweat—are either ontologically neutral (hair clippings) or ontologically repugnant (urine, feces, pus), the opposite of self value. They must be cleansed from the self-image if it is to remain intact (Kristeva 1982). These represent dirt or waste for the self.

Clinical treatments and settings produce another order of waste tissue. Hospitals and clinics routinely take human tissue samples for diagnostic testing, and doctors excise pathological or excess tissue during surgery. Historically, hospitals treat such tissue as "abandoned." That is, the person from whom the tissue has been taken has been understood to have relinquished it, and to have no intention of reclaiming it (Gottlieb 1998). The tissue is tacitly considered to have no value or significance for the patient, an assumption shored up by the common law history of treating tissues outside the body as *res nullius,* matter belonging to no one (Dickenson 2002). It is simply waste, abandoned to the hospital rather than donated to another through an act of informed consent. Waste or abandoned tissue is therefore a third term between tissue gifts and tissue commodities, a category of value largely ignored in Titmuss's account of tissue economies, but one which we argue is central to the way the value and significance of tissues is created and transformed. Waste does not simply add an alternative to these forms of value but instead mediates and informs them in complex ways, as we will explore in the next two chapters.

These two kinds of waste, ontological and clinical, can form the starting point for significant kinds of commercial and epistemological productivity, and often tissues simultaneously embody both kinds of waste value. Valuable genetic knowledge may be abstracted from saliva and hair samples, and hormonal material distilled from urine. Hospitals may sell tumor tissues to cancer researchers, or placentas to pharmaceutical and cosmetic companies. They may use the tissue in their own research laboratories and patent promising cell lines. Most of the human cancer cell lines for sale on the web site of the American Type Culture Collection are derived from abandoned tissue,[1] and the "donors" are unlikely to know about this use of their cells (Andrews and Nelkin 2001). Here we can see that waste material in one context becomes a source of value in another, and waste tissues have historically followed the trajectory from body to clinic to laboratory, and from waste to valuable entity, with various degrees of transformation along the way.

To develop this point further, Cooper (2006), in a far-ranging argument, describes the burgeoning biotechnology industries of the last thirty years as working through the reanimation of waste biological material, the creation of new forms of commercial value from living matter previously considered marginal. While historically hospitals have sold these marginal materials in simple commodity transactions, Cooper suggests that the advent of biological intellectual property regimes in the 1980s reconstituted waste tissues as locales for speculative investment. While nation-states have to varying extents withdrawn from the funding of biomedical research, venture capital now funds patentable research that establishes property rights in the future capacities of reengineered matter. This form of totalizing waste reanimation is, Cooper writes, the engine of the biological knowledge economy, and a major dynamic in post-industrial economies more generally.

However, as we saw in chapter 2, the establishment of intellectual property in human tissues requires the prior dispossession of the donor, either through the process of designating the tissues as abandoned, or through the informed consent procedure, which effectively declares the tissues a form of unimproved waste, valueless until channeled through the circuits of technical and capital transformation. Unsurprisingly, this blatant dispossession is becoming more and more controversial. Tissues once safely regarded as waste—saliva or cancerous material, for example—are today caught up in the biopolitics surrounding the status of genetic information, the right to genetic privacy, and the kinds of protections afforded to donors by informed consent. The social consensus around what constitutes a waste or abandoned tissue is breaking down, so that the economy of waste tissue rehabilitation is becoming more complex and contested.

In the following chapters, we will consider two cases in which the donors themselves challenged the status of their tissues as waste. In chapter 3 we discuss a landmark court case, *Moore v. Regents of the University of California*, which revolved around the contestation of property in waste tissue. The donor, Moore, lost his case, but the judgment tells us a great deal about the logic that informs the political economy of waste tissues and their crucial position in tissue commerce. In chapter 4 we examine the trajectory of an erstwhile waste tissue, umbilical cord blood, revalued by recent biotechnical developments and discoveries. Since the late 1980s cord blood functions both as a gift, circulated by public cord-blood banks, and a form of private, speculative biological investment, managed by a for-profit tissue bank. The private, autologous cord-blood account is, we argue, an innovation in tissue value, which enables parents to invest their children's tissues in the future of biotechnical progress.

3

The Laws of Mo(o)re

WASTE, BIOVALUE, AND

INFORMATION ECOLOGIES

In 1984 John Moore, an Alaskan engineer, filed suit against his former physician, Dr. Golde, Golde's employers (the Regents of the University of California system), and several pharmaceutical companies. In *Moore v. Regents of the University of California* Moore charged that the defendants had effectively stolen his spleen and transformed part of it into a commercially available cell line, from which they were all making large profits. While the defendants did not agree that they had stolen Moore's spleen, they agreed with the basic facts asserted by Moore. In 1976 Moore, suffering from hairy-cell leukemia, had gone to Golde, a medical specialist and researcher at the University of California, Los Angeles. Golde urged Moore to let him surgically remove his spleen. Moore's lawyers later discovered that before making this recommendation, Golde knew that Moore's diseased cells produced unusually large amounts of lymphokines. Lymphokines are proteins used by the body's immune system and are of use and interest to many researchers. However, lymphokines were also notoriously difficult to produce in large amounts, and so Golde saw great economic potential in Moore's cells. If he could create an immortal cell line from his tissue, then he would have created a biological factory for producing large amounts of lymphokines. Such a cell line could be sold commercially.

By at least 1979, Moore's doctors had used material from the excised spleen to create this cell line (originally called the "Mo" cell line, but later renamed "RLC"), and in 1981 established a patent on the cell line (U.S. Patent No. 4,438,032). Golde and his research assistant, Shirley G. Quan, were listed as inventors, and their employers, the Regents of the University of California, were listed as assignees of the patent. The Regents licensed use and production of the cell line to Genetics Institute, Inc. (and later Sandoz Pharmaceuticals), in exchange for stocks and cash. Moore charged Golde, Quan, Genetics Institute, Sandoz Pharmaceuticals, and the University of California with, among other things, failing to provide him with appropriate information (in the form of informed consent disclosures) and "conversion" (that is, the unauthorized appropriation of his property). The Superior Court of Los Angeles County found that Moore had no property rights in his cells and thus that no conversion had occurred. The Court of Appeal of California reversed this decision, arguing that Moore did have a property right in his cells and thus that the defendants had "converted" the cells. The final (split) court decision of the California Supreme Court reversed the appellate court decision, establishing—as the first court had—that Moore had no property right to his cells.

The *Moore* case has been the subject of intense interest on the part of both legal critics and cultural historians. It has been described as exemplary of the paradoxical status of "intellectual property" in an information society (Boyle 1996); as indicative of the vexed role played by conceptions of "dignity" in the age of biocommerce (Rabinow 1996; Rabinow 1999; Mitchell 2004); as a case study in the imperialistic advance of economic value over all other forms of social value (Kimbrell 1997; Gold 1996); as an example of the deconstruction of the purported opposition between gift and commodity systems of exchange (Frow 1997); and as paradigmatic of attempts to understand new forms of biotechnology and humanity by making recourse to old stories of race and nation (Wald 2005).

Moore provides a further explication of the property relations underpinning commercial biotechnology that we began to discuss in chapter 2. The judgments in the case are eloquent statements of the stakes and power relations involved in intellectual property relations in the biotech domain, particularly those surrounding the dispossession of tissue donors in these intellectual property regimes. In our treatment of the *Moore* case, we are particularly interested in the role that ideas of waste played in the various court decisions, and in the process of donor dispossession. Previous commentators have noted, but only in a cursory way, that the majority in the state supreme court discussed at some length the similarities between Moore's cells and human feces, and ruled that Moore had "abandoned" his diseased cells to the "safe hands" of UCLA's infectious waste system. Yet the topic of waste, we suggest in this chapter, did not constitute a puzzling aside in the court's decision but was central to the logic of biomedical innovation that it sought to support. In chapter 2 we noted that informed consent was a mechanism for what Callon (1998) calls "disentanglement": that is, informed consent separates embryos from parents so that embryonic tissue can be transformed into patented stem cells. The category of waste performed an almost identical function in the *Moore* case, enabling the biological and legal separation of tissues from Moore so that an immortalized cell line could be produced.

However, the role of "waste" in the process of disentanglement at play in *Moore* depended upon three earlier, and initially separate, discourses on waste, human tissues, and information flows that unfolded in the United States. The first discourse focused on safety regulations designed to reduce the threat of useless, and potentially infectious, human tissues. In addition, the court implicitly positioned Moore's diseased spleen within the context of another discussion of biomedical waste that dated back to debates about human blood in the 1960s and organ transplantation in the 1980s. This discourse focused on *valuable* human tissues, such as blood and organs, and linked the dissemination of these tissues to the smooth flow of information between management facilities (for example, hospitals and blood banks); the absence of such information flows was purported to produce tissue waste in the form of expired blood and degraded organs. The court knotted these two discourses together by drawing on yet another, though much more recent, discourse on waste that had emerged in the context of hearings that preceded the passage in 1980 of the Bayh-Dole Act. This legislation was designed to reinvigorate "innovation" by assigning patents to corporations rather than the U.S. government, because (so the argument went) assigning them to the government had resulted in a huge waste of innovation. The Mo cell line linked all three of these discourses: it was produced from diseased human tissue; it stood poised to become part of a therapeutic information flow between hospitals and researchers; and it demonstrated the "successful" transformation of federal funding into private property. The intersection of these three discourses on waste in *Moore* provides a vital insight into how contemporary biocommercial research and development in the United States depends upon an understanding of waste as both culturally constructed and structurally necessary.

Moore, Biowaste, and "Safe Hands" When Golde first considered creating a cell line from Moore's spleen tissue in 1978, technologies for cell line immortalization were by no means a new thing. In the first three decades of the twentieth century biological researchers such as Ross G. Harrison and Alexis Carrel had developed technologies for maintaining living tissue outside an organism: Carrel, for example, began a cell line with embryonic chicken fibroblasts which he claimed to have maintained from 1912 to 1946 (Landecker 2000, 55; Squier 2000). By the 1950s a number of "immortal" cell lines had been established, including the well-known HeLa cell line (produced from cervical cancer tissue taken from Henrietta Lacks). However, researchers in the 1960s also discovered that only cancerous tissue could serve as the basis for natural immortalization, and thus many of the noncancerous cell lines previously understood as immortal were in fact contaminated with other kinds of cells. In the 1970s successful techniques for immortalizing noncancerous cells were developed, though it remained considerably harder until the 1990s to create cell lines from noncancerous tissue. Luckily for Golde and Quan, the nature of Moore's illness facilitated their task, and creating the Mo cell line simply required isolating the cancerous cells.

While the cell line technology employed by Golde and Quan was only arguably "innovative," the legal environment in which they operated was in flux. Just as *Moore* began what would be its decade-long journey through the California court system, the U.S. Supreme Court was in the process of fundamentally altering the terrain of biotechnology patent law. A number of bioengineered plants and animal lines had been produced in the 1970s, but patent applications on genetically engineered entities had been routinely rejected by the U.S. Patent and Trademark office. In an attempt to press the issue of the patentability of bioengineered flora and fauna, Anadada Chakrabarty, an employee of the Genetics Division of General Electric and "inventor" of an oil-eating bacterium, appealed the rejection of a patent application that he had originally submitted in 1972. As Stone (1996) notes, Chakrabarty's bacterium seems to have been carefully designed to serve as the basis for a test case for the more general question of animal and plant patents. It was not clear that the engineered bacterium could survive outside the laboratory, a quality which (Chakrabarty and GE hoped) would establish a clear distinction between "natural" and "engineered" organisms.

However, the Patent Board of Appeals ruled that Congress had specifically exempted genetically engineered organisms from patent protection in the Plant Variety Protection Act of 1978, and so denied Chakrabarty's appeal. Both Chakrabarty and the Patent Board commissioner (Sidney Diamond) appealed. The U.S. Court of Customs and Patent Appeals and, subsequently, the U.S. Supreme Court (in 1980) reversed the Patent Board decision, ruling that there was no intrinsic difference between a "composition of matter," which could be patented, and an engineered plant or animal: thus, they concluded, the latter should also be patentable (Stone 1996). Commenting later on the ruling, the U.S. Office of Technology Assessment stated: "[t]he question of whether or not an invention embraces living matter is irrelevant to the issue of patentability, as long as the invention is the result of human intervention" (Rabinow 1996, 131–32). Thus by 1980 the patentability of genetically engineered tissues and organisms was no longer an issue, though the test case had involved a bacterium rather than a human cell.

Nevertheless, the *Moore* case was clearly a vexing one for each of the three California courts asked to hear it. In addition to the scores of pages devoted to the majority opinion of the California Supreme Court, three of the justices wrote their own opinions, one concurring with the majority, one concurring in part and dissenting in part, and one dissenting. The court offered a number of rationales for its holding that Moore had no property rights in the cell line developed from his tissue. The majority held, for example, that the Mo cell line was biologically different from the cells that had existed in Moore's spleen, and since it was Golde, not Moore, who had performed the "inventive labor" to transform the spleen cells into the Mo cell line, Moore could not claim property rights in the cell line. In addition, Moore's claim that he owned his spleen threatened to establish a dangerous precedent: if all research subjects were able to claim such property rights, research would grind to a halt, since the "exchange of scientific materials, which still is relatively free and efficient, will surely be compromised if each cell sample becomes the potential subject matter of a lawsuit" (*Moore v. U. of Cal.* 1990, 162).[1] In any case, the majority opinion continued, body parts in general could not be owned by the individuals from whom they were derived.

This claim about the ownership of body parts forced the majority justices into a discussion of human waste, a topic earlier broached in the Court of Appeal decision to support Moore's property claim. Moore's lawyers, in their appearance before the Court of Appeal, had cited in support of their property claims the case of *Venner v. Maryland* (1976), which concerned the legality of a police seizure of a criminal defendant's feces for evidence. In that case the Maryland Court of Appeals had concluded that a defendant had the right to control the search of his "abandoned" feces. In support of this claim, the Maryland court reasoned that just as people often assert "ownership, dominion, or control" over body parts such as "hair, fingernails, toenails, blood and organs," so too ought one be able to exert these powers over "excrement, fluid waste, [and] secretions" (*Venner v. Maryland* 1976, 498). In *Moore* the California Court of Appeal had accepted this reasoning, and simply added another item—"diseased tissue"—to this list of body parts, holding that individuals must be allowed to exert ownership, dominion, or control over these tissues as well. "A patient must have the ultimate power to control what becomes of his or her tissues," the court wrote, and to "hold otherwise would open the door to a massive invasion of human privacy and dignity in the name of medical progress" (*Moore v. U. of Cal.* 1988, 508). The court noted that human waste such as feces lacked the "dignity of the human cell," which suggested even more strongly that if feces could be owned, then certainly other tissues must be the potential subject of property right as well. "[T]he legal significance of this reference [to *Venner v. Mary-*

land]," the court held, "is the [Maryland] court's statement that it *cannot* be said that a person has no property right in materials which were once part of his body" (*Moore v. U. of Cal.* 1988, 505).

The California Supreme Court disagreed emphatically with this line of reasoning, stating that both Moore's lawyers and the Court of Appeal had mistaken privacy rights for property rights. The majority ruled that Moore's lawyers had been unable to locate any precedent establishing that diseased human cells could be owned by an individual such as Moore. "No party," they wrote, "has cited a decision supporting Moore's argument that excised cells are 'a species of tangible personal property capable of being converted'" (*Moore v. U. of Cal.* 1990, 157 n. 28). Instead, the majority continued, both Moore's lawyers and the Court of Appeal had attempted to use privacy rights to support a property claim: "[l]acking direct authority for importing the law of conversion into this context, Moore relies, as did the Court of Appeal, primarily on decisions addressing privacy rights" (*Moore v. U. of Cal.* 1990, 156). *Venner v. Maryland*, in other words, was about the right of a patient to keep his wastes private, not about the right to "own" his feces. Thus both Moore's lawyers and the Court of Appeal had made a category mistake. "[O]ne may earnestly wish to protect privacy and dignity," the majority wrote, "without accepting the extremely problematic conclusion that interference with those interests amounts to a conversion of personal property. Nor is it necessary to force the round pegs of 'privacy' and 'dignity' into the square hole of 'property' in order to protect the patient, since the fiduciary-duty and informed-consent theories protect these interests directly by requiring full disclosure" (*Moore v. U. of Cal.* 1990, 158).

Golde and the University of California system, the court implied, may have "interfered" with Moore's privacy and dignity, but this did not mean that the interference was best addressed by awarding property rights to Moore. Rather, one could rely on existing fiduciary and informed consent duties to protect privacy and dignity. These duties required that physicians and researchers such as Golde disclose beforehand if they had any financial interest in the tissues or information of their patients and subjects. Golde clearly had not informed Moore properly, but the court contended that this breach could not be resolved by allowing Moore to own a share of the cell line created by

Golde. Both Moore's lawyers and the Court of Appeal, in this view, were laboring under the mistaken belief that feces could be "owned," and sought to apply their faulty logic to tissues such as surgically removed spleens. But, the California Supreme Court held, to allow Moore to own his diseased spleen would be dangerous, and in direct conflict with state statutes that dealt with infectious waste. The court ruled that Moore had "abandoned" his diseased cells when he consented to their surgical removal, and thus agreed to their disposal in the biological waste system of the UCLA hospital facility. This waste system was regulated by Health and Safety Code section 7054.4, designed to safeguard public health by mandating that "recognizable anatomical parts, human tissues, anatomical human remains, or infectious waste following conclusion of scientific use shall be disposed of by interment, incineration, or any other method determined by the state department [of health services] to protect the public health and safety" (Health and Safety Code section 7054.4, cited in *Moore v. U. of Cal.* 1990, 158). The court noted that "virus-infected cells such as Moore's T-lymphocytes fit reasonably within the statute's definition of 'infectious waste'" (*Moore v. U. of Cal.* 1990, 158 n. 32). Public safety required that such dangerous materials be delivered to what it called "safe hands" (*Moore v. U. of Cal.* 1990, 158 n. 33), a description that applied to the UCLA hospital system but not to Moore. Reports on infectious waste published in 1989 and 1990 had revealed that about 2.2 million metric tons a year of medical waste were produced by American hospitals each year, of which 15–20 percent was infectious tissues (Manns 1995, 547, 553 n. 1, citing Rutala, Odette, and Samsa 1989, 1638; Fay et. al 1990, 1494). To allow individuals such as Moore to "own" their infectious cells, the court implied, would make it impossible to insure that diseased tissues made their way to the safe hands that protected public safety.

Yet the majority argument concerning safe hands and public safety was something of a red herring, for Moore was not interested in owning the remnants of his excised spleen: instead he wanted a share of the profits generated from the cell line made from it.[2] Presumably the justices focused on the diseased spleen because they believed that a property claim in the cell line could only be based on an anterior property claim in the excised spleen itself. However, their argument

went, since the public statute dealing with biowaste "eliminates so
many of the rights ordinarily attached to property that one cannot
simply assume that what is left amounts to 'property' or 'ownership' "
(*Moore v. U. of Cal.* 1990, 175), then one need only show that Moore
could not own his spleen to show that he could not own the cell line
made from the spleen. However, as Justice Mosk noted in dissent, just
because a statute "eliminates many of the rights ordinarily attached to
property" does not mean that no rights are left. Mosk provided an
extensive list of the different rights attached to different kinds of property: a fish sportsman can give his catch away, but cannot sell it; a
person "contemplating bankruptcy may sell his property at its 'reasonably equivalent value,' but he may not make a gift of the same property"; and so on (*Moore v. U. of Cal.* 1990, 177 n. 9). In other words,
Health and Safety Code section 7054.4 of the State of California might
regulate the property claims of individuals on tissues, but it did not
necessarily preclude those claims. Moreover, Mosk noted, the majority
certainly was not suggesting that public safety required denying *all*
ownership in the excised cells, because presumably the defendants'
property rights in the Mo cell line depended on precisely the same
anterior property right that the Court denied to Moore. The UCLA
infectious waste system, in other words, allowed someone to own
Moore's spleen, but not Moore.[3]

The ontological instability of the object under question—Was this
case about Moore's spleen or the "Mo" cell line?—complicated considerably the relationship between waste and property. This point had
been articulated in a dissent to the earlier Court of Appeal decision, in
which Judge George wrote that even if one accepted the definition of a
diseased spleen as property, "the question arises whether this 'property' was worthless as a matter of law 'at the time of the conversion'
[that is, when it was removed from Moore's body] and whether there
was any further 'loss' as the 'proximate result' of the purported conversion. . . . It was only after defendants expended great effort, time, and
skill that—in my opinion—plaintiff's spleen acquired *any* of the char-
acteristics of property, at which time this diseased organ became trans-
muted from human waste into patentable blood cell-lines" (*Moore v.
U. of Cal.* 1988, 537). George likened Moore's spleen to "raw material,"
which "evolved into something of great value only through the un-

usual scientific expertise of the defendants, like unformed clay or stone transformed by the hands of a master sculptor into a valuable work of art" (*Moore v. U. of Cal.* 1988, 537). In the Court of Appeal the point of dispute between the majority opinion and George's dissent was whether Moore's spleen and the Mo cell line were related as points along an ontological continuum—a position that might allow property rights held at one point to be transferred to another—or rather, as George claimed, an ontological gulf existed between the two forms of tissue.[4] In George's dissent, we find the same logic of value that we explicated in the discussion of embryonic cell line patents in chapter 2. Here too donated tissue is presented as valueless matter, transformed into valuable property through the formative power of a technical idea, the "intellectual" content of intellectual property.

The California Supreme Court, while it did address the ontology of the various tissues, sought to make an end run around this issue by suggesting that the property claims of Golde, Quan, and the University of California depended on their status as "safe hands" that protected public safety, a status that Moore did not have.[5] Yet the court made clear that the connection of Golde, Quan, and the University of California to these safe hands did not depend solely—or even primarily—on their connection to a hospital capable of incinerating or interring infectious human remains. Rather, it depended on their location within a scientific-legal climate, or "ecology," that connected basic research to the corporate production of therapeutic medical products for the public.[6] The court argued that the development of therapeutic products from basic research required a complicated ecology of information and tissue flow between university researchers and corporate developers. The first condition of this ecology was a free flow of information and tissues between basic researchers such as Golde and his colleagues at UCLA and other university institutions. "At present," the court wrote, "human cell lines are routinely copied and distributed to other researchers for experimental use, usually free of charge" (*Moore v. U. of Cal.* 1990, 162). The progress of science, in other words, required an efficient and unrestricted flow of information and cell lines from institution to institution. Yet the progress of therapeutic medicine required that this basic science be transformed into specific products and therapies that could be released into the field of corporate market competition. The court suggested that corporations would be unwilling to accept the responsibilities of shepherding research into products unless they had an unambiguous property right in cell lines or information. Thus, in addition to the free flow of scientific information and tissues between basic researchers, "progress" required that some tissues and information become the exclusive property of corporations. The court linked these two realms of flow through an image of exponential research growth: "[t]housands of human cell lines already exist in tissue repositories," and these repositories themselves "respond to tens of thousands of requests for samples annually"; these research requests, in turn, resulted in an ever-expanding array of therapeutic products that benefited everyone (*Moore v. U. of Cal.* 1990, 161).

The court contended that awarding Moore property rights in the Mo cell line would destroy both the free flow of scientific information and the economic incentives that led to medical therapies. Giving Moore property rights in the Mo cell line would also destroy the flow of medical therapies to the public, the court argued; "the theory of liability that Moore urges us to endorse threatens to destroy the economic incentive to conduct important medical research" (*Moore v. U. of Cal.* 1990, 162). To hold corporations liable anytime they used a cell line developed without the permission of the "donor" would make companies reluctant to develop any therapies at all.[7] The court acknowledged that granting property rights in cells might "enforce patients' rights indirectly," but suggested that the cost of such protection was too high: "to extend the conversion theory would utterly sacrifice the other goal of protecting innocent parties" (*Moore v. U. of Cal.* 1990, 161).[8] Allowing Golde and Quan to own the Mo cell line facilitated the system that created biomedical value out of infectious waste products. Granting Moore property rights in his cells, by contrast, would not only contravene the infectious waste statutes of California, but—far more important—would *create* waste, by uselessly sacrificing innocent parties.

The court thus positioned the safe hands of the UCLA biological disposal system in relation to two kinds of waste. The first was actual biomedical waste, such as Moore's diseased spleen. The UCLA system allowed such waste to be safely mined for value, because doing so enabled a physician such as Golde to transform *potentially* useful bits of waste into value, while at the same time disposing of infectious matter that was truly useless. At the same time, though, the court invoked a much more virtual form of waste: that is, the waste of lives and talent that would occur in the future if patients such as Moore were allowed to own their own tissues and thereby stall the flow of research and commerce. It was the specter of this latter form of virtual waste that compelled the court to award property rights to Golde and withhold them from Moore. The category of waste thus allowed the diseased spleen to be disentangled from Moore and transformed into a property that could be manipulated by Golde and other researchers.

Precedents: Waste and Information Flow in Earlier Tissue Economy Debates Virtual waste had played an important part in previous discussions of tissue economies in the United States, but the court's opinion in *Moore* subtly altered the valence of several terms in the discourse. In the blood bank hearings of the 1960s and organ transplantation hearings and legislation of the 1980s, witnesses had claimed that tissue donations would ensure the free flow of information and the therapeutic use of tissues, while commodification of blood and organs would waste valuable tissues and lives. In the *Moore* decision, by contrast, the need for donation was limited to one point of the system—namely, Moore—while subsequent commodification was presented as necessary if waste was to be avoided.

As we noted in part I of this book, in the blood banking debates that took place in the United States in the 1960s, "donation" was constantly linked to the free—and therapeutic—flow of information. The Federal Trade Commission had angered a number of doctors and hospital administrators by arguing that banked blood should be considered a commodity, since it differed materially from blood as it was found in the body (citrate was added to banked blood). It also argued that since blood was a commodity, then informal communications between physicians about the regulation of inter-institutional blood supplies could be considered "conspiracy." Yet most of the medical witnesses called to testify during three days of congressional hearings contended that defining blood as a commodity would impede flows of information about blood supplies, which would in turn produce massive biomedical waste. They suggested that the problems of blood typing and the relatively short shelf life of blood militated in favor of measures to increase the amount of information shared between physicians, blood banks, and hospitals. Dr. Charles Wheeler noted that "[w]hen pathologists meet, there is an exchange of all types of scientific information. They may exchange information about blood sources just as there may be an exchange of information about varieties of heart medicine . . . but this unanimity of opinion does not represent the result of a conspiracy" (U.S. Congress 1964, 133). Many witnesses painted pictures of the unpleasant effects of stalled information flows, describing, for example, rare blood type stocks that languished in one hospital though they were desperately needed in a hospital nearby, simply because no information flowed between the two institutions. "Stalled" information created holes in the blood circulation infrastructure, which caused severe wastage of blood resources. Donation systems, many of these witnesses claimed, were better because they produced less waste. From the perspective of these critics of for-profit blood banking, the problem with defining blood as a commodity rather than as a gift was that it impeded information flows and thereby produced waste.

As we will explore at greater length in chapter 6, congressional debates in the 1970s and 1980s concerning organ transplantation revolved around the topic of stalled information flows in almost identical fashion. The problem of organ donation was consistently positioned as a problem of "supply" and "demand," but only a very few witnesses advocated solving the problem by commodifying whole organs. Instead witnesses and bill sponsors such as Representatives Henry Waxman and Albert Gore Jr. maintained that there was no real organ supply problem, but simply a failure to distribute information about this option to people donating organs, as well as a failure to coordinate information about organs and donors between hospitals and organ donation groups.[9] Gore and other witnesses suggested that should these information flows be facilitated, the supply of organs would increase as potential donors became real donors by signing donor cards, and organ waste could be minimized through a centralized computer network that determined the most appropriate matches between organs and recipients. The discussion of organ transplantation,

like the earlier discussion of blood banks, was influenced by the specter of waste, and this possibility was tied to the collapse of information
flows and the commodification of human tissues.

In the *Moore* case the California Supreme Court drew selectively on
these earlier debates about blood and organs. As in the earlier debates
about blood and organs, the free flow of information was held up as a
fundamental requirement for protecting public health. Without gifts
of money and tissues from the public to researchers, the court contended, and without the free flow of information and tissue samples
between researchers, the public would cease to receive improved medical products and therapies. Yet the court departed from these earlier debates, suggesting that tissue samples (for example cell lines)
had to operate according to both the regime of the gift *and* the regime
of the commodity. The gift economies that existed between the public and research institutions, and among research institutions themselves, were not enough to ensure public health. They had to be supplemented by a commodity economy that turned gifted tissues into
property.

The court's divergence from these earlier discourses on tissues and
the gift can be traced to another discourse that purported to explain the
connections between information, waste, and the gift-commodity distinction: namely, the public debates that prepared the way for the
Bayh-Dole Act of 1980 (P.L. 96-517). This bill had its proximate origins in a series of government reports in the 1970s, widely discussed
in the national media, that seemed to show a decrease in innovation in
the United States relative to its trading partners, particularly Japan.
Journalists noted that "increasing competition from countries such as
Japan and West Germany was taking business away from American
industries" (Rensberger 1972, 29), a trend that could be tracked by the
"declining growth rate of the US economy," the "worsening balance of
trade," and the "decreasing number of US patents issued to US inventors and an increase in patents issued to foreign inventors" ("Patent
Bill Seeks Shift to Bolster Innovation" 1979, § D, 8). Rather than
attribute the slip in the economic preeminence of the United States to
changes in either the world economy or the production infrastructure
of countries such as West Germany and Japan, many commentators
suggested that a national "innovation crisis" was to blame (Sullivan

1976, 44; McElheny 1976, § D, 1). Jerome D. Wiesner, president of the Massachusetts Institute of Technology, charged that the "pace of innovation in American technology is slowing down," and this sentiment was echoed a few months later by Dr. Simon Ramo, the chairman of President Ford's Committee on Science and Technology (Wiesner cited in Schmeck Jr. 1976, 12; Sullivan 1976, 44). Concern about the status of innovation in the United States persisted into the next administration, as President Carter initiated his own study "to find out why innovation by private industry is in the doldrums" (Kelmenson 1979, § F, 14). Members of Congress responded to these concerns through a series of hearings and bills devoted to the topic of scientific and business innovation, and especially to the topic of patent reform.[10] By 1978 the Bayh-Dole Bill had become the locus of these congressional hearings.

Waste quickly emerged as one of the dominant themes of the Bayh-Dole hearings. One of the bill's co-sponsors, Senator Birch Bayh, Democrat of Indiana, set the tone for the hearings by opening them with the claim that "talent responsible for the development of numerous innovative scientific breakthroughs each year" was "going to waste as a result of bureaucratic red tape and illogical government regulations" (cited in Stevens 2004, 95). The most serious source of waste, Bayh claimed, was the government's ability to appropriate the patent on any invention produced with the help of federal funding. Witnesses appearing before congressional panels on government patent policy repeatedly painted a picture of inventions "wast[ing] away in government storerooms, benefiting no one" (U.S. Congress 1980a, 551). Many witnesses repeated the claim that by the 1970s the federal government owned over 28,000 patents, only 5 percent of which had been licensed to a private corporation for development (U.S. Congress 1976, 8).[11] Howard I. Foreman, deputy assistant secretary of commerce for product standards, claimed that the "products of the inventive genius of the Nation are not unlimited," and thus "must be conserved and nurtured just like our timber reserves, our oil deposits, our mines and our farmlands. We cannot afford to allow them to become decayed or eroded through lack of use" (U.S. Congress 1976, 14). The root cause of Japanese and western European economic success, these witnesses implied, was the faulty patent system of the United States, which allowed the federal government to appropriate, and thereby waste, the "products of the inventive genius of the Nation." The decay and erosion of national inventive genius could not be measured directly, of course, and so the specter of the future loss of inventions functioned as a virtual image, intended to motivate lawmakers to create conditions in which "undiscovered" inventions could be discovered and put to public use (U.S. Congress 1976, 82). To fix the system, they argued, inventions should be placed into the hands of those who would not squander them, but would instead provide for their conservation and cultivation.

Many of the witnesses were aware that it might seem unfair to grant to individuals and corporations the exclusive patent rights for inventions produced with the support of federal tax money. One critic suggested that the proposed changes in patent law might well "constitute one of the greatest giveaways in our history," but others contended that patents multiplied the social benefits of innovation (U.S. Congress 1980a, 463).[12] The chairman of one hearing encouraged a witness to defend the claim, presented in an earlier hearing, that "the benefits to the public generally from the development of an innovation and its commercialization, was a multiple of . . . some 20 to 30 times the benefits which accrued to the developer or inventor of a particular invention" (U.S. Congress 1976, 80). The witness happily complied with this request, arguing that the "personal gain" which accrued to Chester Carlson, inventor of the Xerox machine, "is by no way to be compared with the amount of gain to the employees, the stockholders in Xerox, the many people throughout the world, the industry, the people, the Congressman's office, all of us who use the Xerox-type invention" (U.S. Congress 1976, 81).

To counter government waste and the loss of "inventive spirit," witnesses posited a fundamentally speculative understanding of innovation. Many implied that the United States stood on the edge of an abyss, into which it would fall should its industries seek to compete with other nations by simply making cheaper or better goods. The lesson to be learned from the Japanese success in developing semiconductors (invented in the United States) was that true economic dominance depended on being at the forefront of constant change. Witnesses and legislators placed their bets on the future; only by constant development of new products could the United States survive economically. What precisely would be produced by companies in the United States in, say, fifteen years was uncertain, but that was precisely the point: if these companies and legislators had no idea what was around the innovation bend, then neither did Japan or the countries of Western Europe. The Bayh-Dole hearings articulated what we would call a "formal" speculative logic: that is, while the specific content of future innovation was unknowable, the legal structures outlined by legislators were designed to ensure that innovations, whatever they might be, were constantly channeled into economic growth. Innovations that did not come into being, or that languished in government warehouses, were a form of waste that the United States simply could not afford.

Bayh-Dole passed in 1980 and significantly changed the relationships between federally funded research institutions and private corporations. The waste purportedly produced by federal control of patents had been replaced by a system of aggressive patenting by public and private research institutions. Large research universities—the major recipients of federal funding—were the first to appreciate the potential profits to be made from the change in patent policy, and medical research became an especially important component of university patent portfolios.[13]

While it is not entirely clear whether the Mo cell line patent was developed with the help of federal funds, it certainly benefited from Bayh-Dole: the act allowed the majority justices to link an understanding of biomedical waste developed in blood and organ debates to claims about virtual waste produced by faulty patent regimes. The Mo cell line itself *must* be owned, the court held, for it was only as a potentially profitable piece of property that it would be propelled out of the university. However, it could not be owned by just anyone, but only by those individuals or groups that were (in the court's estimation) committed to generating ever-new forms of tissue and informational property. Just as witnesses in the Bayh-Dole hearings had argued that encouraging patents on federally funded inventions would result in an exponential increase in social benefits, the majority in *Moore* painted an almost identical picture of the expanding social benefits of a cell line patent, with thousands of human cell lines already in tissue reposito-

ries responding "to tens of thousands of requests for samples annually," leading eventually to many new therapeutic products. The
court suggested that this sort of exponential growth required an extremely careful calibration of property rights, since any misstep would
destroy the whole system. More precisely, this system of exponential
social benefits required that property rights emerge at the nexus of
two kinds of flows: on the one hand the free flow of information characteristic of science, and on the other the profit-directed flows of
time and energy characteristic of entrepreneurship. While scientist-
entrepreneurs such as Dr. Golde stood within this nexus, Moore—an
entrepreneur but not a scientist—stood outside the circle of value
generation, and thus could not be awarded property rights.[14]

Peddlers, Recycling, and Biovalue   In a curious way Golde's relationship to waste revived elements of earlier industrial networks of rubbish sorting. In an illuminating history of waste in the United States,
Susan Strasser traces the role of peddlers in the construction of industrialism, noting that rather than simply provide consumers with
objects, peddlers also gathered consumer "waste," such as rags or
hair, to sell to the paper and wig-making industries. "As the United
States industrialized," Strasser writes, "the same wholesalers, peddlers, and general storekeepers who introduced new manufactured
goods to households acted as the middlemen in the marketing process
for waste materials" (Strasser 1999, 73). This two-way flow of goods
and waste required a discriminating eye on the part of these middlemen, who had to distinguish between saleable and unsaleable "waste"
(this was especially true of peddlers, who had to transport the waste
that they received from consumers on their backs). In the 1970s and
1980s, as the economy of the United States made a shift from Fordist
to post-Fordist models of production, physicians such as Golde found
themselves occupying a position quite analogous to that of the earlier
wholesalers and peddlers. Physician-researchers were middlemen in
two senses: they "sold" new therapeutic technologies to patients and
their insurance companies, and at the same time they used their discriminating eyes to pick out nuggets of potential value from their
customers' wastes, which they then shuttled back to firms such as
Sandoz Pharmaceuticals for further development.

Yet even as Golde's function within a shifting economy mirrored that of late-nineteenth-century peddlers in the early stages of industrialism, the telos of waste had shifted in ways that transformed the modes of exchange between consumers and middlemen. Golde was a speculative peddler: unlike the linen rags collected by nineteenth-century peddlers, the wastes that Golde sold to Genetics Institute could not be processed directly into consumer products. Rather, the Mo cell line was designed to unlock the multiple potentials of other biological tissues, which would in turn result in a cascade of therapies and drugs. Moore's property claim, the California Supreme Court concluded, threatened to block the exponential growth of innovation upon which the economy of the United States depended. Thus, where nineteenth-century consumers had sold or bartered waste to middlemen, late-twentieth-century consumers such as Moore were required to give, not sell or barter, their waste products.

The court's image of exponential growth was itself an index of much larger and more fundamental shifts in the financing of medical and pharmaceutical research and development, and the legal framework in which it took place. As Robin Blackburn has outlined in *Banking on Death* (2002), investment capital from pension funds in the late 1980s and 1990s moved into increasingly speculative ventures, a process which fueled the dot.com and biotech "bubbles" of the mid- to late 1990s. In a very literal sense, the economic future of many employees of corporations in the United States was tied directly to the success of speculative biotechnology; as Melinda Cooper notes, "the so-called new economic growth of the late 90s—characterized by the spectacular rise of digital and life science technologies in the US—would not have been possible without the speculative investment provided by the mobile savings of (mostly US based) salaried workers, funneled onto the capital markets by increasingly powerful institutional investment and mutual funds" (Cooper 2006). In her analysis of changes in bio-financing, Cooper sees Geron (founded in 1990) as typifying this shift, noting that while the company offers "little more than the hope of future revenues from its patent portfolio," it nevertheless continues to attract investors (Cooper 2006). It does so, she argues, in large part because its patents on stem cells seem to promise a future wealth of innovation and property claims. The developmental biologists Markus

Loeffler and Christopher S. Potten have written that "stemness is not a property but a spectrum of possibilities," and Geron's patents are designed to encourage, and at the same time economically exploit, the numerous biological possibilities of its cell lines. Cooper observes, "the only thing sustaining Geron's faith in the future is its claim on the intellectual property rights of all future inventions using its products" (Cooper 2006). The *Moore* case demonstrates the extent to which these shifts in patterns of finance were dependent upon an intellectual property regime in the United States that since the 1980s has proved itself increasingly willing to extend patent protection to cell lines, genes, and gene sequences.

What is perhaps most striking about the role of waste in *Moore* is the extent to which the court itself seems to have anticipated recent sociological theories about waste and value. As John Frow notes, the sociology of value begins with the proposition that "value is a process, a movement, a cycle, rather than a quality of things or a structure of cotemporal relations"; that is, "value is an effect of the circulation of objects *between* regimes of value" (Frow 2003, 35). The court in *Moore* fully subscribed to this view, since it did not claim that Moore's spleen was intrinsically valuable—or, for that matter, intrinsically valueless—but only that its status as value or waste depended on its movement between institutions such as "the public," "the research institution," and "the corporation." The court was able to propose this "constructivist" understanding of waste and value precisely because it was opposed to the system of "reciprocal" or "balanced" exchanges which purportedly underpin stable systems of value (Frow 2003, 35). Instead the court argued that the creation of value depends on an intrinsically unbalanced system, in which public "waste" could be converted first into private value and then into public value by means of biomedical therapies and products.

Waste, Biovalue, and the Laws of Mo(o)re The *Moore* case has been the subject of an extraordinary number of critical discussions in the fields of law, sociology, anthropology, cultural studies, and bioethics, but as several commentators have noted, the significance of the case lies primarily in its value as an index, more than as legal precedent. The direct impact of *Moore* on subsequent court decisions appears to be relatively slight. While several decisions have cited *Moore*, and some of these citations occurred in relatively high-profile cases, it is nevertheless true, as Sealing notes, that "[i]n the decade since it was decided, Moore has generated a large number of citations but has not often been followed" (Sealing 2002, 761).[15] Yet *Moore* has been symptomatic of the legal and economic changes establishing the basic terms in which contemporary biocommerce is understood.

Opinion about what exactly *Moore* represents varies widely, depending on the commentator. For authors writing for popular audiences, the case has often been the locus of outrage against the injustices committed by "corporations" and a legal system stacked in their favor (see for example Kimbrell 1997). More sophisticated analyses have stressed that *Moore* exposes the extent to which strategies of appropriation once reserved for the third world—for example, the perceived right to appropriate *terra nullius* (empty land)—are being extended to the citizenry of first-world countries (see for example Shiva 1997; Harry 1995). Yet *Moore* is especially important for exposing the central role played by waste in producing biovalue. As we have noted throughout this book, biovalue is premised on what we might call "speculative biology"; that is, biovalue refers not to the stable and known properties of tissues but to the capacity of tissues to lead to new and unexpected forms of value. As *Moore* illustrates, the capacity of tissues to generate new and unexpected properties does not inhere entirely in the flesh itself. Rather, tissues achieve this capacity only within very particular, speculative, social "ecologies." Unlike the steady-state systems imagined by proponents of blood and organ donation, which rely on reciprocal exchange and which produce known quantities and types of therapeutic products (blood categorized by type and organs linked to immunological profiles), speculative social ecologies are designed to facilitate the emergence of *new* properties and tissues. These speculative ecologies employ many of the conceptual categories employed by earlier tissue economies. The category of the gift, for example, was as important to the justices in *Moore* as to earlier advocates of blood and organ donation, and the ecology outlined by the *Moore* court sought to minimize some forms of biomedical waste, just as the proponents of gift economies of blood and organs had. Yet despite these surface similarities to earlier tissue economies, the speculative social ecology outlined in *Moore* altered radically the valence of these terms.

These altered valences are particularly visible in the category of waste, for while majority justices deplored some forms of virtual waste, they were explicitly committed to the active production of what we might call "constitutive waste": that is, waste that is the precondition for producing "the new." The court suggested that Dr. Golde was able to pick out the potential value of Moore's lymphokine-overproducing cells only because, in his capacity as a speculative physician-peddler, he could distinguish the difference between Moore's spleen and the majority of (useless) spleens he had removed from other patients. Exercising this capacity for recognition was no simple task, since Moore's spleen cells were not in and of themselves valuable but only manifested *potential* value; they were waste, in other words, that promised value. One could discern the promise of value, the court suggested, only against an otherwise homogeneous field of waste. The homogeneity of this field was threatened by patients such as Moore: if they were allowed to bargain over the value of their cells, discerning potential value in the field of waste would become impossible. Waste was thus the category linking Moore to an imagined community and annulling the possibility that he could maintain property rights in his excised tissues. In their role as constitutive waste, Moore's donated (rather than owned) tissues were part of the basis for the fiscal and biological health of the body politic.

4

Umbilical Cord Blood

WASTE, GIFT, VENTURE

CAPITAL

We saw in chapter 3 that John Moore was prevented from establishing a property right in his cells, in part because the cells were considered waste. As diseased, infectious material, the spleen cells were deemed by the court to have no negotiable value for him, and his claim of ownership was denied. In this chapter, we investigate another example of tissue until recently considered waste—umbilical cord blood. As in chapter 3, our interest is in the relationship between the persons (mother and child) from whom the tissue arises, and the value of the fragment itself. Over the last fifteen years or so, blood derived from the umbilical cord has been transformed from a waste product, at the disposal of the hospital, to a clinically valuable substance, useful for the treatment of serious blood disorders. In this process of re-valuation, the ontological status of umbilical cord blood has changed as well. While it was once considered an abject tissue, designating neither mother nor child, it is now deemed a significant fragment of the infant.

In both the United States and the United Kingdom, parents may donate their child's cord blood to public banks that distribute it according to clinical need. They may also bank it privately. Private cord-blood banks have created a commercially and culturally innovative, although clinically questionable, form of biological property—the private cord-blood "account." As we will see, this form of biological property structures the relationship between owner and fragment somewhat differently from the commodity form pursued unsuccessfully by Moore. It does not pose this relationship as one between proprietor and alienable asset, negotiable on a market, but as one between investor and investment. The private cord-blood account is organized as a source of biological investment material that may be deployed in a number of ways to create and protect the health of the investor. The account holder is not a vendor but an entrepreneur. In this chapter we will investigate cord blood's itinerary from clinical waste to venture capital, and consider its future as a model for other emergent kinds of personal biological investment capital.

Cord Blood and Bone Marrow   Umbilical cord blood has become therapeutically valuable tissue over the last fifteen years because it can substitute for transplanted bone marrow in treating blood disorders. Since the 1970s bone marrow transplants have been used to rebuild the patient's blood system as part of the treatment for leukemia, immune deficiency, aplasia, and genetic metabolic disorders.[1] Bone marrow is the source of the body's blood system and is rich in hematopoietic (blood-generating) stem cells. While transplanted bone marrow is the first choice of treatment for these serious conditions, bone marrow is a highly entangled and recalcitrant tissue, difficult to source, donate, and match. It is not amenable to the forms of standardization and circulation that characterize more bankable human tissues like blood products or cell lines.

Like solid organs, bone marrow is immunologically inflexible. Finding donors is extremely difficult because their bone marrow must have very precise HLA (human leukocyte antigen) matching with the patient's tissues. The number of possible combinations of HLA alleles is very high, with only a 25 percent chance that a sibling will have sufficient compatibility for a safe donation, and only a one in four hundred chance for an unrelated person (Kline 2001). If relatives are not suitable, a patient may seek a donor through the national and international bone marrow donor registries, set up during the 1980s to facilitate transplant. Currently nearly 8 million people are registered worldwide, a small number compared to the possible HLA combinations.[2] It may take months to identify and locate possible donors, who must visit a clinic for tissue typing and health assessment before scheduling a donation. Often no suitable donor can be found. An incorrect tissue match is potentially fatal. A remnant of the patient's immune system may destroy the graft, leaving the patient without functional immunity to infection. Alternatively, the graft may reject the entirety of the patient's tissues in a phenomenon termed graft-versus-host disease, which in its most severe form produces liver failure, gastrointestinal bleeding, and death. Even well-matched sibling donors carry a 20 percent risk of some degree of graft-versus-host disease (Kline 2001).

In addition to these tissue-matching difficulties, the donation of bone marrow is onerous. Donation involves hospitalization and an invasive harvesting procedure. The donor is anaesthetized, and about a liter of bone marrow is syringed from the hip bones or sternum, often from several points. After the procedure the donor stays in the hospital overnight, and may need a blood transfusion.[3] Donors take between three days and three weeks to recover fully from the procedure. Thus bone marrow donation is comparable to the more invasive forms of live tissue donation—egg, kidney, liver lobe. Donors may find themselves in a painful, ongoing relationship to the recipient. They may be asked to donate repeatedly to the same patient if first or subsequent treatments fail. At the same time, donors cannot make occasional donations as blood donors do, because the procedure is arduous and risky, and a particular donation may never be needed. Currently the U.S. National Marrow Donor Program has four million registered donors, but only facilitates 130 donations per month.[4] The donation is not readily separable from the donor, and therefore donation is only undertaken when there is a definite recipient. Registers of potential donors must suffice, rather than banks of the material itself.

Umbilical cord blood, the hundred or so milliliters (about half a cup) of blood retained in the placenta and cord after birth, is a more tractable and disentangled source of hematopoietic stem cells. The existence of hematopoietic stem cells in cord blood was identified thirty years ago (Knudtzin 1974), but no clinical use was made of this knowledge until the late 1980s, when the first allogenic cord blood transplant was used to successfully treat a boy with Fanconi's anemia, using his newly born sibling's cord blood (Gluckman, Broxmeyer, Auerbach, et al. 1989). Since that time umbilical-cord-blood transplants have been used to treat an ever-growing range of malignant and nonmalignant conditions—aplastic anemia, sickle cell anemia, thalassaemia, genetic immunodeficiency syndromes, myelogenous and lymphoblastic leukemias, neuroblastomas—generally when a suitable bone marrow donor cannot be found. Cord blood is much more accessible than bone marrow. It is harvested during birth, when the cord is already quasi-external to both the maternal and infant bodies. It is also much easier to match with a recipient because it is "naïve." That is, cord blood is not strongly characterized immunologically and does not mount a strong response when faced with tissue from another body. Hence cord blood does not have the stringent HLA matching requirements of bone marrow, and even poorly matched tissue does not carry the same danger of graft-versus-host disease (Kline 2001). Currently cord-blood transplants are used primarily to treat children, as the small quantity available for harvest is about ten times less than the quantity of bone marrow, making cord blood more suitable for patients with smaller body weight. Researchers are trying to develop methods to expand stem cell mass in vitro so that larger volumes can be transplanted (De Haan et al. 2003).

Umbilical cord-blood transplantation is still considered an experimental procedure, and only 2,500 transplants had been carried out worldwide by mid-2003 (Jana 2003). Cord-blood transplants have about the same relapse and success rate as bone marrow transplants (Sirchia and Rebella 1999). The small amount of tissue available means that cord blood is slower to engraft than bone marrow, leaving the recipient vulnerable to infection for a longer period than with a successful bone marrow graft (Laughlin, Barker, Bambach, et al. 2001). However, the burgeoning interest in stem cells and stem cell technologies, discussed in chapter 2, has carried over into this field as well. Research projects are under way around the world to improve the utility of cord blood for transplant and to identify new clinical applications. Commentators habitually predict a great clinical future for umbilical cord-blood treatments.

From Garbage to Gold   Cord blood is thus a substance that has recently acquired clinical value. Journal articles about umbilical cord blood frequently emphasize a dramatic transformation from valueless waste product, the detritus of the birthing process, into a valuable therapeutic substance. An article in the Research News section of *Science*, entitled "Umbilical Cords: Turning Garbage into Clinical Gold," begins, "Ordinarily, one of the least significant products of a birth is the umbilical cord: the cord is usually just discarded with other detritus. But recent research is changing all that. What was discarded has become valuable—indeed priceless to many children with leukemia, and perhaps in the future to children with AIDS and autoimmune diseases, such as diabetes and rheumatoid arthritis" (Thompson 1995, 805). An article in *Scientific American* relies on a similar narrative of value generated from garbage. "After cutting the cord . . . the doctor usually tosses [the umbilical cord] into a stainless steel bucket with the rest of the medical waste bound for incineration. But more and more physicians and parents are realizing the value of what they used to regard as merely birth's byproduct" (Kline 2001, 42). A recent interview in *Newsweek* with Stephan Sprague, one of the first adults to be successfully treated with an umbilical cord-blood transplant, makes a plea for recognizing the value of the umbilical cord: "I had end-stage leukemia and they were telling me to get my affairs in order," he says. Six years after his stem cell transplant he remains cancer free—and disturbed that most cord blood ends up as medical waste, not in public banks: "If some anonymous mother hadn't decided to donate, I wouldn't be talking to *Newsweek* right now" (cited in Jana 2003, 57).

In these accounts the umbilical cord has been transformed from detritus to "clinical gold," and the problem now is to regularize hospital obstetric and waste management procedures to ensure that this revaluation is recognized. However, we argue that this new valuation of the umbilical cord is not simply a creation of value from nothing but a transformation in *kinds* of value. Waste tissue, as we noted earlier, is tissue deemed to be of no value or interest to the person from whom it originates. Waste tissue is therefore defined in terms of a presumed relationship between person and fragment. As the cultural critic Walter Moser notes, the term "waste" implies a certain relationship between fragment and totality: "Waste is often fragmentary, partial, residual in relation to a totality that would have preexisted it. The French *déchet*—singular, nominative—conveys this sense better perhaps. The separation of part from whole is usually one of the genetic pre-conditions for the existence of waste . . . waste is that part which has been actively detached (torn, ejected, expelled) from a whole and subsequently cast off and excluded: refuse" (Moser 2002, 86–87).

Following Moser, we consider that the zero degree of value assumed by the articles cited above is in fact an assessment of the value of the tissue for the person from whom it originates. It is understood as waste *for them*, a fragment of self that has been detached and caste off. It has lost its ability to designate self, except in a negative way, as a dangerous or disgusting excrescence, something that threatens bodily integrity and must be removed and contained. However, for hospitals and clinics that have the right of disposal, waste tissue has considerable commercial and epistemological value, as we demonstrated in chapter 3. This was true of the placenta and umbilical cord before their clinical value was established, and is still true in hospitals that do not have cord-blood collection programs. Hospitals routinely sell placentas to cosmetics companies that use them in a variety of skin creams (Andrews and Nelkin 2001), and cords and placentas are sold to pharmaceutical companies for the extraction of albumin, an ingredient in many pharmaceutical products. Companies like Pasteur-Merieux Sérums et Vaccins in France collected eight million placentas annually in the early 1990s (Nau 1993). Here classification as waste makes such tissues available for profitable forms of recycling.

Abandoned tissue also makes a valuable contribution to medical knowledge, in part because it is free of the administrative encumbrances associated with informed consent procedures. The Royal College of Physicians has stated that the "use of anonymised left-over tissue for research is a traditional and ethically acceptable practice that does not need consent from patients or relatives, and need not be submitted to a research ethics committee" (cited in Hurley 1995, 23). The recently proclaimed Human Tissue Act of 2004 in Britain specifies that the use of such delinked tissue for research will continue to be exempt from consent requirements, as long as the proposed research has received ethics approval.

Umbilical cord blood has been used extensively in this kind of de-linked research over the last thirty years. Cord-blood samples have been used to monitor epidemiological distributions of diseases and toxins. For example, they have been used as an indicator of biological lead levels in residential areas (Gershanik, Brooks, and Little 1974). Unlinked, anonymized testing of umbilical cord blood has been used to track the prevalence of HIV infection in certain populations (Fiala 2000). Cord blood or tissue can be used to build up tissue samples in research biobanks. Umbilical cord material is currently being collected for genetic research through the North Cumbria Community Genetics Project (Chase et al. 1998). Umbilical cord blood has also played a valuable diagnostic part in pediatric medicine. Doctors can assess the health of an infant by using cord blood rather than blood samples (Vawter 1998). Cord blood can also provide a source of autologous blood transfusion for ill or premature infants (Ballin 1995).

It is precisely because hospitals did not discard umbilical cord blood, but instead circulated it through clinical and laboratory sites for over thirty years, that researchers recognized it as a source of hematopoietic stem cells. In addition to epidemiological, genetic, and pediatric medicine, umbilical cord blood was used in basic hematology and immunology research. Knudtzin's identification of hematopoietic stem cells in cord blood (Knudtzin 1974) ensured that scientists interested in fundamental blood biology studied cord blood throughout the 1970s and 1980s. Some researchers assessed the quantities of stem cells in cord-blood samples and realized that the concentration was similar to that of bone marrow (Broxmeyer, Douglas, Hangoc, et al. 1989). This finding brought cord blood to the attention of clinicians dealing with blood disorders and the difficulties of obtaining bone marrow donors (Broxmeyer et al. 1990).

In sum, cord blood has had a complex significance and positive value for hospitals and laboratories, a value facilitated by its status as clinical waste. Cord blood was redeployed, with little in the way of bureaucratic or bioethical obstacles, to various experimental, research, and commercial contexts where it was put to a multitude of uses. As waste, cord blood has been particularly mobile, able to move from a potentially unprofitable context (disposed of in hospital incineration systems) to a multitude of profitable ones, generating institutional income, research prestige, and useful pure and applied biomedical knowledge. The kind of opposition intended by the rhetoric of "garbage into gold," the opposition between the valueless and the valuable, is hence misleading. The umbilical cord may have been designated "waste," but as we discussed earlier, waste is frequently a covert or latent form of value, all the more valuable for being unacknowledged.

Clinical Value The identification of its clinical applications, and the demonstration of efficacy in the first successful transplant (Gluckman, Broxmeyer, Auerbach, et al. 1989), precipitated a dramatic reclassification of the value of cord blood, in two interlinked ways. First, cord blood migrated rapidly from waste to therapeutic substance. Its value is no longer measured against other abandoned yet useful clinical wastes—biopsy tissue, urine samples, and so on—but instead against other life-saving tissues—organs, blood, and above all bone marrow. Both bone marrow and cord blood are highly valued because they preserve the lives that count as the most precious, those of children. They treat a feared disease, leukemia, and other serious conditions. In this new hierarchy, cord blood often ranks above bone marrow. The flexibility and durability of cord blood are routinely contrasted to the intractably entangled, particular nature of bone marrow. Many articles offer assessments like the following, from an editorial in *Contemporary Obstetrics/Gynecology*: "Umbilical cord blood offers many advantages over unrelated donor-derived bone marrow as a source of stem cells for an affected sibling, including a higher likelihood (25%) of an HLA match and ready availability. Moreover, when used by unrelated third-party recipients, umbilical cord blood derived stem cells seem to confer advantages in rates of engraftment and reduced graft-versus-host disease even if there are one or two HLA loci mismatches. The latter phenomenon may reflect the cells' relative immaturity and the higher proportion of stem cells in an umbilical cord specimen than in bone marrow. Indeed, preliminary results are sufficiently reassuring that, in my opinion, the [U.S.] government should aggressively fund not-for-profit public umbilical cord blood stem cell banks" (Lockwood 2002, 8).

Cord blood also habitually ranks above bone marrow because of the relative ease of the harvesting procedure. This provides both a bioethical and an immunological benefit in the estimate of many commentators (Lockwood 2002; Burglo, Gluckman, and Locatelli 2003; Bourque and Sugerman 2000; Kline 2001). As we saw, the donation of bone marrow is quite onerous, involving registration, blood testing, hospitalization at short notice, general anaesthesia, and the pain and risk involved in any invasive procedure. In contrast, cord blood is donated at the time of birth and causes pain for neither mother nor infant. Physical risk is generally considered minimal, although some bioethicists are concerned that staff members may have their attention diverted from the mother and child during the process of collecting cord blood (Vawter 1998; Comité Consultatif National d'Ethique 2002).

The relative ease of donation means that in principle at least, cord-blood donors are more plentiful than bone marrow donors, and cord-blood banks should be able to access a spectrum of ethnic groups with particular genetic profiles (Lockwood 2002). Moreover, because cord blood is a substance that can be banked for ten years or more, routine collection allows the accumulation of a range of HLA tissues over time. The London Cord Blood Bank has established a collection in which over 40 percent of the donations were from non-European groups, whereas the British Bone Marrow Registry lists only 2 percent of its donors as non-European (Armitage et al. 1999). As tissue is already donated, tested, characterized, and located in a particular site, tissue matching is much more rapid than the procedures for bone marrow: "Identifying a suitable unrelated bone marrow donor is a time consuming process that takes an average of four months. . . . In contrast, cord blood is readily available from a bank's freezer and has already undergone viral testing and tissue typing. An umbilical cord blood match can be made in as few as three or four days, which can spell life or death for someone who is already immunodeficient and at high risk for a fatal infection" (Kline 2001, 48).

So in the clinical hierarchy of transplantable tissues, cord blood is more valuable than bone marrow with regard to ease of harvest, immunological flexibility and spread of HLA combinations, cost in risk, time, and pain to the donor, and speed of matching and delivery. It benefits from the heightened value generated by tissue banking—that is, the detailed control over harvesting, storage, and circulation that it affords. It is these qualities that lend to it the quality of clinical "gold," the most valuable of substances.

Ontological Value   Cord blood value has been transformed in a second way: through the reversal of its abject status, its status as waste for the person. The protocols associated with abandoned tissue, specifically the absence of informed consent, become both clinically and bioethically problematic when applied to therapeutic tissues. Its clinical revaluation brings cord blood under the protocols and regulations governing anatomical gifts in the United Kingdom[5] and human tissues in the United States.[6] Moreover, its clinical value inheres in the particular genetic markers and health status of the blood, qualities that derive from both the maternal and infant bodies linked by the umbilical cord. While the cord blood has the same tissue type as the infant, maternal health influences its quality, specifically the presence or absence of infectious agents like HIV, hepatitis B and C, cytomegalovirus and syphilis, and genetic conditions like immune system or blood disorders.[7] In hospitals with collection programs, cord blood can no longer be considered abandoned. Parents must donate their child's cord blood through an informed consent procedure. Bourque and Sugerman describe the transition: "When research on cord blood was just beginning, many researchers assumed that informed consent was unnecessary because umbilical cord blood was waste to be discarded. However, as umbilical cord blood showed therapeutic promise, the need arose to obtain sensitive health-related information about the donor, and the calculus shifted to requiring informed consent" (Bourque and Sugerman 2000, 67–68).

  Thus parents may donate their child's cord blood to a public bank, where it will be used for an allogenic tissue donation. However, private cord-blood banks offer to parents a quite different way of managing the relationship between their child and the cord-blood fragment. In the following pages we will consider these different protocols for ordering cord blood.

Cord-Blood Banking   Cord-blood banking, like all tissue banking, produces clinical outcomes through the manipulation of biological time. Cryopreservation is a way to preserve the hematopoietic potential of the stem cells. Like embryonic stem cells, cord-blood stem cells are valuable because they partake of the generative capacity of the prenatal body in both its maternal and its fetal aspects, its striking ability to produce and renew organized tissue. Banking these tissues—that is, freezing them—removes them from the flow of historical and biological time, and preserves them so that their potential can be realized at a later date. Banking turns the *generative* capacities of the prenatal body into *regenerative* capacities, the capacities to revitalize the sick or aging postnatal body. In this respect cord blood stem cells increasingly partake of the same dream of a regenerative body evident in embryonic stem cell claims (Waldby 2002a), the dream that every biological loss can be repaired.

There are two institutional approaches to preserving the potential of cord blood: public banks use one, private banks the other. Public banks primarily accept allogenic donation, although some accept autologous donations from families at risk of hereditary blood conditions. The New York Blood Center set up the first allogenic cord blood bank in the United States in 1993, and the London Cord Blood Bank was set up in 1996. These are now among a number of public cord blood banks in the United Kingdom, North America, and other nations in the developed world.

Public banks create clinical value for cord blood through the redistributive processes of the public tissue gift economy that we have discussed at length. They focus particularly on the need to accumulate tissues. Blood banks that handle peripheral blood, the kind circulating through the body, try to keep supply and demand in relative equilibrium, because many fractions of peripheral blood are perishable. Cord blood stores well for long periods, so banks focus on building up supply and maximizing the spectrum of tissue types available to patients. The London Cord Blood bank aims to collect and store ten thousand units, including samples from the diverse ethnic groups living in the United Kingdom (Armitage et al. 1999). At the time of writing, a bipartisan Cord Blood Stem Cell Act was before the U.S. Senate, designed to create a network of cord-blood banking centers with an inventory of 150,000 units. Public banks also participate in international registries that aim to find tissue matches overseas if no national match can be found.

Private cord blood banks create a different kind of value through a very different accumulation strategy. They sequester cord blood in a personal account, withholding it from all forms of allogenic circulation. The first private cord-blood bank, that of the Biocyte Corporation, was set up in Connecticut in 1993 (Holden 1993), and now private cord-blood banks operate throughout the United States, Europe, and Asia.[8] Private banks lease autologous banking facilities to parents, who pay an annual fee to bank their child's cord blood for future use. Private banks recommend autologous storage as a way to avoid the vagaries of the public cord-blood matching process. Private banking, they claim, ensures that the child will have access to a source of perfectly matched tissue on demand, and so protects the child and possibly other family members against the risks of developing otherwise untreatable conditions. The web site of the Mount Sinai Hospital Cord Blood Program states, for example, "The majority of children will fortunately never need the stored cells. However, some children will have their health severely affected by such genetically transmitted blood diseases as Thalassaemia, Sickle Cell Disease, or some forms of anaemia or immunodeficiency disease. Other children will be stricken with such cancers as childhood leukaemia, malignant lymphoma or neuroblastomas. While childhood cancer is fortunately a rare event, it is the leading cause of death in children between the ages of one and fourteen."[9]

Private cord-blood banking has attracted the condemnation of virtually all medical professional and bioethical bodies.[10] The consensus among these bodies is that cord-blood banking for personal use is not warranted by the very low risk that any given person will develop a blood disorder treatable by cord-blood transplant. In 1997 the American Medical Association issued a consensus statement that described autologous cord blood transplant as an unproven treatment and the marketing practices of private cord blood banks as needing close attention (American Medical Association, Working Group on Ethical Issues in Umbilical Cord Blood Banking 1997). The American Academy of Pediatrics issued a policy statement in 1999 stating that parents should not store their children's blood for future use unless there is evidence of family predisposition to leukemia or other blood conditions (Kline 2001). A scientific opinion of the Royal College of Obstetricians and Gynaecologists condemned the practice of private cord-blood banking:

> It is difficult to estimate the likelihood that an individual directed dona-tion would be used. This applies especially given that many of the pro-jected usages of stem cells remain speculative and subject to research yet to be done. There is also the presumption that treatment advances involving stem cells will be readily available on the N H S. One commer-cial storage provider estimates that likelihood of a child developing a disease that could be treated by stem cells by the age of 18 years as around one in 300–400. Although stored cells might also be used by other family members, this figure seems a gross overestimate of the probability that a stored cord sample will ever be used. One bank in the U S A has to date issued only two units out of 10,000 stored, although this figure may rise with time. At present, it is not possible to conclude that storing cord blood for one's child will not be of value, although the likelihood that it would ever be used is very low. (Royal College of Obstetricians and Gynaecologists 2001, 2)

The French national bioethics commission opinion on cord blood banking (Comité Consultatif National d'Ethique 2002) notes that au-tologous donation is contraindicated in many of the conditions listed at the private cord blood banks' web sites: "In the case of a genetic disease, it is difficult to understand how such cells could be useful to the patient concerned, since the cells would be carrying the same mutation, unless some presently unknown effective gene therapy were to emerge. For some of these genetic diseases, allogenic grafts, from a related or an unrelated donor, could be indicated. For many haematological diseases, remission or cure also relies much more on allografts than on autografts. For a wide range of leukaemias, the immunological reaction capacity of allogenic cells to factors carried by the leukaemia cells, have a beneficial effect: i.e.' the graft versus host leukemic cells reaction. Autologous cells would not have this effect" (Comité Consultatif National d'Ethique 2002, 3).

In other words, the autologous capacity to regenerate oneself is not clinically desirable in all cases: in genetic conditions, it is precisely the mutated nature of the autologous tissue that is problematic, and in some other blood disorders the effects of allografts are clinically beneficial. Moreover, current autologous stem cell treatments are mainly used for adults and drawn from the patient's peripheral blood. The report notes that any technical innovation that would potentiate cord blood would also potentiate peripheral blood, so that it would be unnecessary to resort to preserved cord blood in any case.

Despite this concerted condemnation, the market for private cord-blood banking services is growing each year (Saywell 2003). Very few studies have investigated the reasons why parents use private banking. In a recent Canadian study of women's attitudes to cord blood donation, Fernandez and colleagues (2003) found that 86 percent of the 443 respondents preferred public cord-blood banking, while 14 percent preferred private banking. Those who preferred private banking stated that it was a good investment for the child, and that they felt obliged to secure their child's cord blood in case of future need. Advocates of public cord-blood banking believe that parents who elect to use private facilities are simply misled by the rhetoric of the private banks. However, in what follows, we want to consider other possible explanations for the attractions of private cord-blood banking. In particular, we want to scrutinize the meanings of autologous cord blood as an "investment." As we will see, private banks do not transform cord-blood waste into clinical gifts, as public banks do, but into biological venture capital.

Biological Investment   We believe that private cord-blood banking creates a new permutation in the relationship between tissue fragment and self. It effectively creates a new form of biological property, one not adequately encompassed by the concepts of either gift or commodity. Rather, the private cord blood account creates a legal relationship between person and tissue fragment that negotiates some of the aporias opened up by contemporary tissue economies. In particular, it addresses the paradox created by the non-commodifiable status of the body for the subject, combined with its status as an open source of biological material for commercial interests. Frow, commenting on the *Moore* case, describes this paradox in the following terms:

> The Moore case sets up two alternative ways in which I can formulate my relationship to my body. In the first, I have a property right, which means that others cannot appropriate parts of my body without my

consent, but also that I have the right to sell all or part of my body. In the second, I have no property right; I can't alienate it, but it has become a commons to which others may lay claim. In both cases, one property right pushes out another. The aporia stems from the central place occupied in liberal thought by the necessary link between self-possession (the form of the person) and property (the commodity form). The classic definition of the category of self-possession . . . is Locke's: "Every Man has a *Property* in his own *Person*. This no Body has any Right to but himself." This self-possessing subject is both the foundation of all other property rights, and the prototype of those things that cannot be alienated in the marketplace. (Frow 1997, 160–61)

While John Moore's case came to grief on this paradox of liberal self-possession, the private cord-blood account creates a form of property that resolves an element of this tension. It does so both technically and contractually. The account leases facilities to the account holder and manages the technical aspects of harvesting and storage; and it creates a legal relation of possession between the unit of cord blood and the account holder. The form of possession that the account creates is novel in the contemporary field of human tissue biopolitics because it severs questions of property from the questions of commodification taken up in the various critiques discussed earlier. It effectively avoids the gift-commodity dichotomy that largely structures the field of bioethical debate around human tissues. The account and its contents are constituted as the property of the account holder, but they do not partake of the commodity form—they have no legal exchange value and are not negotiable for price on a market. The value of the cord blood for the account holder resides precisely in its not being alienated, in its perpetual retention, because of its self-regenerating capacities. The account constitutes cord blood as a possession, yet an inalienable possession (Weiner 1992), a fragment detached from the self that nevertheless belongs to it irrevocably. For those who open private cord-blood accounts, the value of their fragment is entirely lost if it is either given as a gift or exchanged as a commodity. The account provides a way to preempt the claims of others on the fragment and preserve its potential for the future self. At best the account may be held as a form of family property, opened by parents on behalf of their child and potentially shared among family members, who have a higher chance of a tissue match.

In public banks, the value of cord blood is allogenic; its clinical usefulness arises at the point of redistribution, when it is transferred from one person to another. However, the private account allows depositors to retain exclusive control and use of their cord blood, on the grounds that its value is primarily *autologous* and *autopoietic*; that is, each account can remake a part of the account holder's body. Banking the tissues privately, diverting them from allogenic networks of gifting and redistribution, is a way to coordinate the self-generative capacity of the cord blood with the aging bodies of account holders. It allows them to live in a double biological time. The body will age and change, lose its self-renewing power, and succumb to illnesses of various kinds. The banked fragment, frozen and preserved from deterioration, retains its negentropic, autopoietic capacity. If need arises, it can literally remake a crucial part of the account holder's body: the blood system.

The private cord blood account is thus a form of property whose value is oriented toward the biological future, both the future health of the account holder and, as we will see, the future of biotechnology more generally. It is this future orientation that qualifies the cord blood as an investment rather than an inert possession with a stable value. The marketing strategies of private cord-blood banks emphasize both the prudential and the speculative investment value of a private account. In its prudential aspect, a private cord-blood account is organized according to the neoliberal principles of private insurance, which offers personalized risk-management services as a hedge against the uncertainties of the future. Public cord-blood banking works through the collectivization of health risk management, its distribution throughout the population on the grounds of capacity and need. Private cord blood banks use risk segmentation, unpooling, and personal risk-management strategies (Ericson, Barry, and Doyle 2000). Private banks play up the uncertainties of the public system, the possibility that no donation is exactly right for *you*, and liken private banking to a form of insurance. For example, the Mount Sinai Hospital Cord Blood Program states that banking cord blood provides "biological insurance: painlessly obtained, immediately available, perfectly matched cells for your child."[11] Lifebank Cryogenics Corporation states that it "offers families biological insurance. Our facility stores the valuable umbilical cord blood (for the families [*sic*] exclusive use)."[12] A private cord-blood account offers the client a form of biological security not obtainable in standard life and disability insurance. These latter forms substitute a capital value for bodily loss, whereas the biological insurance offered by private cord-blood banking is a way to repair bodily loss itself, or at least certain kinds of loss, those associated with diseases of the blood.

Private cord-blood accounts are also marketed as a form of speculative investment, one whose use-value might multiply in unforeseeable ways in response to new biotechnologies. This aspect of cord-blood banking has gained particular impetus from the field of regenerative medicine. Regenerative medicine enhances the body's self-repair capacities through the use of growth factors like recombinant EPO (Erythropoietin), used to enhance the production of red blood cells; tissue engineering, which involves, for example, the culture and growth of a person's own skin to treat burns; and stem cell research, which encompasses the use of embryonic stem cells, "adult" stem cells like nasal epithelial cells (Mackay-Sim 2004), and cord blood stem cells. Hematopoietic stem cells do not display the pluripotent versatility of embryonic stem cells in current technical conditions, nor can they be cultured into cell lines.

Nevertheless, considerable research is currently under way to find better ways to enhance cord blood and bone marrow stem cell capacities and confer on them the same aura of potential that embryonic stem cells have. Research is being conducted into ways to culture cord blood stem cells so that they can be "expanded" in the same way as embryonic stem cell lines (Egan 2000) and to induce transdifferentiation into multipotent stem cells, rather than stem cells committed solely to the production of the blood system (Anderson, Gage, and Weissman 2001). Bone marrow cells are currently being used in small clinical trials around the world to rebuild cardiac tissue after heart failure, for example (Hirschler 2003).

Private banks increasingly emphasize this open-ended nature of stem cell research. Ron Penny, the director of Cryosite, the first private cord-blood bank set up in Australia, stated in a recent interview: "if you look at the material we have produced carefully, you will see that we have not over-emphasised the use in leukaemias. We emphasise much more the long term future applications of the earliest form of adult stem cells."[13] An interview with the scientific staff at CORD, a private cord blood bank in California, makes a similar point: " 'What happens . . . when, say, diabetes can be cured with a cord blood stem cell transplant?' asks Cohen. 'In another five years, I believe cord blood would become more commonplace.' But if and when it does become commonplace, there would be no way of going back and collecting cord blood samples from those [already] born. 'You miss the chance if you decide to throw out the cord blood,' said Dr. Joy Traille, lab director at CORD" (Raghunathan 2001).

The Mount Sinai Hospital program points to the possibility that gene therapies may make use of cord blood stem cells in the future. "New gene therapies are being developed that may depend on the use of cord blood stem cells to treat diseases that are presently difficult to treat or incurable."[14] Parents are urged to seize the moment and create a private cord blood account for their child, in an act of open-ended hope in biotechnical progress. In particular, they invest in the possibility that cord blood will achieve the plasticity of embryonic stem cells, which have apparently endless, pluripotent possibilities for multiplication and recapacitation. As Cooper (2006) notes, the rhetoric around stem cells, and indeed the material organization of immortalized stem cell lines, constantly affirms the open-ended possibilities of these new entities. Stem cells acquire their value in a speculative, virtual realm, in projections of possible therapeutic applications and possible new repertories of activity and agency. Those who hold private cord-blood accounts take an active stake in such future biotechnical developments, and the possibility that they will progressively enhance the value of their cord-blood investment in innovative ways.

Among the medical organizations critical of private cord-blood banking, the French national bioethics commission makes the most explicit link between different models of banking and the formation of social order and citizenship. Its report states:

Preserving placental blood for the child itself strikes a solitary and re-strictive note in contrast with the implicit solidarity of donation. It amounts to putting away in a bank as a precaution, as a biological preventive investment, as biological insurance, whereas the true useful-ness of the action in the present state of scientific knowledge, may be negligible . . . There is major divergence between the concept of preser-vation for the child decided by parents and that of solidarity with the rest of society. Systematic auto-preservation, unless for exceptional medical reasons, is a denial of donation and an obstacle to the creation of banks for others which would require very costly prior immunogenetic iden-tification . . . It appears that systematic storage of placental blood for exclusively autologous uses, in the present state of medical science, would be illusory, and more closely connected to market objectives than to therapy. (Comité Consultatif National d'Ethique 2002, 7–8)

The commission appeals to the generosity and social sense of cord-blood donors, their duty of citizenship and their desire to avoid a poor investment—to waste cord blood by saving it inappropriately. In the tradition of Titmuss, they assert that the relationship between person and biological fragment is not simply one of clinical interest, but has broad implications for the shape and order of the polity, its collective or privatized ethos. They appeal to a particular order of medicalized subjectivity, a particular kind of bioethical citizenship associated with a state commitment to universal and redistributive medical care. How-ever, their appeal competes with the appeal of a more recent dynamic of medical subjectivity, exemplified by private cord-blood account holders, for whom new medical technology and health consumer ser-vices are a means of transforming their body into a strategic enter-prise. Novas and Rose (2000) describe this neoliberal medical subjec-tivity as a positive response to the devolution of medical care from the state to private providers. Health is less a matter of collectivized citi-zenship and identification with the nation, and more a relationship of active, critical stake holding and consumption, organized around "the norms of enterprising, self-actualising, responsible personhood that characterize 'advanced liberal' societies, and with the ethics of health and illness that play such a key role in their production . . . these new forms of subjectification are linked to the emergence of complex ethical technologies for the management of biological and social existence, located within a temporal field of 'life strategies' in which individuals seek to plan their present in the light of their beliefs about the future that their genetic endowment might hold" (Novas and Rose 2000, 488).

This neoliberal medical subjectivity is oriented toward the entrepreneurial maximization of future health, an enterprise enabled by burgeoning markets for various kinds of presymptomatic testing (for diabetes, cholesterol, genetic conditions, neurological conditions), preventive pharmacology (anti-aging drugs and vitamins), and enhancement medicine, which addresses not illness but perceived bodily deficiencies (obesity, metabolism, sexual performance). Thus it is deeply invested in new medical technologies and their proposed futures for the body. As Novas and Rose (2000) observe, this mode of subjectification is oriented toward norms of personal responsibility, risk aversion, and informed decision making, as opposed to the norms of participation in collective population health invoked by the CCNE report.

We argue that private cord-blood banking is one of the more innovative technologies that call this mode of subjectivity into being. Its form of investment appeals to these norms of entrepreneurship, risk management, and collaboration with the future of biotechnology. Doubts about the current clinical value of a cord-blood account are outweighed by its potential speculative value, as a source of autologous tissue that might be profitably deployed in relation to new stem cell or genetic techniques. In the words of one parent, "I think it's quite clear that this technology is moving very quickly, and for not a huge amount of money, in fact quite a small amount of money it's a good punt."[15] This calculus, it seems to us, is the reason why the clinicians' warnings go unheeded by a number of cord-blood donors, who elect to use private facilities.

Private accounts allow the account holders to deploy their children's tissues in productive ways without giving them away, losing them to commercial interests, or being placed in a position of indebtedness to another donor. If, as Frow (1997) argues, the social relations that order gift and commodity economies are "intimately bound up with forms of the person," then the novel form of self-possession proffered by private cord-blood banking points decisively toward such an emerging mode of medical subjectivity.

It seems likely that private cord-blood banking might form something of a prototype for other kinds of autologous tissue banking, as the field of regenerative medicine expands. For example, recent dental research suggests that parents should keep their children's baby teeth, as the pulp may eventually be used to regenerate dental tissue in the adult mouth.[16] Therapeutic cloning, now in its earliest experimental stages, is likely to produce a market for private cell line banking if the technology becomes routine. Cloned pluripotent cell lines promise to be the ultimate self-renewal technology, but the high cost of establishing viable lines is likely to exclude the practice from national health budgets and render it the prerogative of the wealthy. The steady aging of populations in the OECD nations creates a large potential market for the possibilities of regenerative biology. As Neilson points out, this potential market is currently motivating much biotechnical research: "There can be little doubt that the intensity of capital investment in this sector, which now drives the economy of certain subnational regions (such as the Boston-Cambridge area in the United States), relates to the expectation of high returns as new technologies of rejuvenation become marketable to an aging population" (Neilson 2003, 181). Private autologous issue banking services may well expand in ways that are responsive in both a positive and a negative sense to the shape of this sort of biocommerce. Excluded from the commercial wealth created by intellectual property rights in tissues, holders of autologous tissue accounts will nevertheless be able to benefit if even some of the possibilities predicted for regenerative medicine and stem cell technologies are realized in clinical applications. If as private citizens they cannot claim commercial wealth in their own tissues, they can nevertheless transform their bodies into a source of venture capital invested in technological innovation.

PART III

Biogifts of

Capital

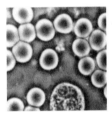 In the first two parts of this book we focused on institutions of tissue exchange that embraced the rhetoric of the gift, even as they often departed from its "spirit" as outlined by Mauss and Titmuss. Thus we considered autologous blood donations, which positioned blood deposits as private accounts rather than communal donations; the UK Stem Cell Bank, which employs the form of the gift primarily as a means of strategically managing the potential conflict between private and public good; the *Moore* case, exemplary of the power of commercial biotechnology and state investment policy to classify human tissues as gifts so that they might be transformed into commodities; and autologous cord-blood banking, which allows parents to use the form of the gift to open personal cord-blood accounts for their children. In all of these examples, we were interested in how the rhetoric of the gift was linked to, and often transformed by, the logic and language of speculative practice. While the values of national communal cohesion described by Titmuss often still served as a point of reference for these new forms of tissue gift exchange, the possibility of "future returns" has come to dominate the institutions of tissue exchange themselves.

This uneasy alliance between the language of the gift and the model of speculative return has inspired two responses in the last two decades. A number of commentators, worried that market relations are overwhelming gift models of exchange, have sought to theorize models of the gift and "common property" that are capable of incorporating the biocommercial imperative for growth and innovation. This move is itself part of a larger interest, first evident in the late 1960s and early 1970s, in the ways that informal norms operate in some geographically bound commons to prevent the "tragedy of the commons" that Garrett Hardin described in his well-known essay of the same name (Hardin 1968; Ostrom 1990; Bromley 1992; Ecologist 1993). More recently legal scholars, anthropologists, and indigenous-rights activists have sought to position the commons—as well as related notions such as "public domain"—as a source of innovation; without the commons, these critics contend, there will be no raw material from which to innovate (Litman 1990; Boyle 1996; Lessig 2001; Shiva 1997). While concepts of the commons and the public domain are generally intended to encompass far more than the tissue economies that are the subject of this book, these claims for the innovative capacities of the commons have become relevant to the circulation of body parts in two ways. First, since the 1970s blood, organs, and medical services more generally have been described in terms of the commons—that is, as a form of common property (Hiatt 1975; Fox and Swazey 1992; Tietzel 2001). Second, to the extent that forms of human tissue are deemed intellectual property—as are stem cell lines, for example—the relationship of these forms of property to the "intellectual commons" becomes a pressing issue (a relationship emphasized in *Moore*).

Yet even as the last two decades have seen an increasing interest in models of the commons, other commentators have urged policymakers to abandon the gift model completely and allow "the market" to dictate flows of human body parts. This appeal was exemplified by Justice Broussard's dissent to the majority opinion in the *Moore* case, in which he wrote that there was no valid reason to bar Moore from profiting from his rare cell line. Calls for market solutions to the problems of tissue exchange have been especially pronounced in the area of human organs, as proponents advocate "compensated gifting" and "futures markets" in kidneys, lungs, and livers (Schwindt and

Vining 1986; Cohen 1989; Blair and Kaserman 1991; Erin and Harris 1994).

While defenses of the gift and the commons have often originated from the political "left," and calls for market solutions from the "right," it is important to recognize that there is often considerable overlap in the stated goals of both commons and market advocates. For example, proponents of the public domain and the intellectual commons often cite innovation as a fundamental value protected by a strong commons, and many of these advocates employ modes of intellectual property specifically to protect the public domain (Boyle 1996; Lessig 2001). In addition, many proponents of the commons believe that at least for certain goods, a commons enables more efficient forms of exchange than a market. While this contention is reminiscent of that by Titmuss (1997) that blood donation systems were far less wasteful than market systems, proponents of the commons maintain that because gene sequences and cell lines are essentially informational products, and thus nonexclusive forms of property (that is, many people can own copies), they enable, and demand, different regimes of use and ownership (Boyle 1996).

Even as advocates of the commons have sought to appropriate the language of the market, market advocates frequently justify their preferences in terms generally associated with the gift. Market proponents have argued, for example, that commodification produces forms of social justice promised, but not delivered, by gift systems of exchange. As we noted in chapter 4, the justices in *Moore* translated the logic of the Bayh-Dole legislation into these terms, arguing that collective health depended upon the competitive forces of the market. However, where the justices' arguments still relied on an implicit gift economy, recent advocates of organ markets contend that donation systems of organ exchange produce cruel (and unnecessary) suffering for patients on organ waiting lists (Blair and Kaserman 1991).

In the next two chapters we focus on two of these "turns" to markets and capital as a way to secure the benefits formerly promised by the donation. Chapter 5 discusses two corporate bodies, PXE International, a patient advocacy group devoted to developing therapies for the genetic disease pseudoxanthoma elasticum, and Affymetrix, a for-profit manufacturer of genetic testing devices. Each group exhibits surprising allegiances. Where one might expect PXE International to lobby against gene patents, in fact it has patented the gene that codes for pseudoxanthoma elasticum. And where one might expect Affymetrix to support gene patents, it has instead lobbied for "open source" genetics. Both case studies underscore how the relationship between profit, community, and health is being reconfigured in the age of speculative biology. In chapter 6 we examine recent calls for legalized markets in human organs, situating these proposals in the context of both the history of organ transplantation in the United States and the recent interest in speculative, regenerative therapies.

5

Commodity-Communities

and Corporate Commons

Court cases such as *Moore*, and developments such as for-profit tissue banking and gene patents, have concerned and in many cases outraged lay and academic commentators. Their concerns have often taken the form of critical studies of biocommerce, some developed from vaguely humanist positions (Kimbrell 1997; Andrews and Nelkin 2001), some from legal positions (Boyle 1996; Gold 1996), others from the perspective of indigenous rights groups (Shiva 1997), and still others from poststructural positions (Frow 1997; Rabinow 1999; Wald 2005). In the last decade many of these diverse theoretical perspectives have found a point of common concern and interest as the prospect has arisen of establishing a "biomedical commons" that would protect certain kinds of human tissues, and information about tissues, from commodification. This interest in a biomedical commons is part of a more general interest in establishing an "information commons" that would protect many kinds of information, ranging from computer code to literary works. As the anonymous author of the Duke Law School newsletter noted recently, advocates of such a development range "from distinguished scientists, software engineers, and gene-patenting experts, to appropriationist musicians, historians and literary scholars," a direct consequence, as the legal scholar James Boyle notes, of the recognition by "people from astoundingly different intellectual backgrounds and fields" that intellectual property legislation is "something that is now dramatically affecting" their work.[1] Advocates of both the biomedical commons and the more general information commons seek to establish national and international institutions and legislation that will protect certain forms of tissue and information from commodification, and create an economy of "free" circulation of these tissues and information among research communities. Some supporters present the biomedical commons as a moral good, capable of protecting human dignity in the face of the sort of "bio-prospecting" that characterized *Moore*, while others present it as a pragmatic imperative, a necessary step in ensuring the continued circulation of research tissues and information. This goal of free circulation was heavily emphasized in the joint statement on human genome research issued on 14 March 2000 by President Bill Clinton and Prime Minister Tony Blair. These two leaders claimed that "unencumbered access to this information will promote discoveries that will reduce the burden of disease, improve health around the world, and enhance the quality of life for all humankind."[2]

Yet this application of the notion of the commons to biomedicine has been complicated by the recent development of new corporate structures that have an interest in circulating tissues and bioinformation. On the one hand, corporations such as Affymetrix (which develops genetic testing devices) have joined the call for creating a biomedical commons; on the other hand, patient rights groups such as PXE International have promoted genetic patent rights as the only means to the equitable sharing of information for the cure of some diseases. Both developments are in some sense surprising: one might expect a corporation such as Affymetrix to fight against the notion of a commons, while patient rights groups seem likely to be staunch advocates of the free flow of information. While the addition of companies such as Affymetrix to the roster of groups supporting the commons might indicate a happy convergence of corporate and human rights interests, the parallel development of intellectual property interests by groups such as PXE International suggests that perhaps these reversals simply dramatize the paradoxes plaguing the intersection of the human body and intellectual property regimes in the present moment.

In this chapter we argue that these two cases illustrate a fundamental paradox of the biomedical commons. Many advocates of the biomedical commons contend that the gift economy characterizing the commons is the precondition of all innovation; without such a commons, and its gifts, there can be no innovation. In this view, all commodities based on patents and copyrights depend on the gift; the gift is logically and temporally prior to the commodity. Affymetrix has embraced precisely this claim, arguing that its patents depend on the existence of a research gift community. Yet the case of PXE International highlights an alternative understanding of these relationships: the basis of its gift community, PXE claims, is the commodity. From this perspective the commodity is logically and temporally prior to the gift. This conflict of interpretations emphasizes what John Frow has described as the "entwinement" of gifts and commodities, such that pure forms of either are impossible (Frow 1997, 124). However, it also emphasizes the increasing importance of innovation and productivity to the supposed distinction between two two categories. At stake in this discussion, in other words, are the conditions necessary for the creation of biovalue. While specific commentators may disagree about the relative contributions of the gift and the commodity to the development of biovalue, all parties agree that biovalue is *the* fundamental value to be protected.

Scarcity and Excess, Regionalism and Cosmopolitanism: Contemporary Theories of Commons   Recent interest in a biomedical commons and an information commons is at least in part a response to an increase in interest since the 1960s in land-based commons. At the same time that Titmuss was defending communal forms of blood distribution, British labor historians of the 1960s and 1970s were researching the process of enclosure that had destroyed most traditional commons in the seventeenth and eighteenth centuries.[3] This historical interest was paralleled by efforts to revalue traditional local commons, as well as efforts to create "global commons" of resources such as the seas, Antarctica, the atmosphere, and outer space. Theorists have attempted to understand and define small-scale local commons (most located in the developing world) not as atavistic remnants of outdated production methods but as sites of production and distribution grounded in an understanding of land use which "provide[s] sustenance, security and independence yet . . . typically does not produce commodities," and where the "relevant local community"—not a national or corporate body—decides questions of land use and access (Ecologist 1993, 7–8). The anonymous authors of *Whose Common Future? Reclaiming the Commons* suggest that " 'Commons' implies the right of local people to define their own grid, their own forms of community respect for watercourses, meadows or paths; to resolve conflicts their own way; to translate what enters their ken into the personal terms of their own dialect; to be 'biased' against the 'rights' of outsiders to local 'resources' in ways usually unrecognized in modern laws; to treat their home not simply as a location housing transferable goods and chunks of population but as irreplaceable and even to be defended at all costs" (Ecologist 1993, 12).

Much of the current literature on contemporary land-based commons also contests the claim that it is an inherently unviable form of land distribution. That latter argument received its most famous formulation in "The Tragedy of the Commons" (1968), in which Garrett Hardin argued that all commons dependent upon finite material substances, such as land, would inevitably be exhausted by "overgrazing," since each grazer would look only to his own interest and not to the community needs (Hardin 1968). Proponents of contemporary land-based commons have noted that Hardin's scenario assumes a neoliberal "self-interested" subject and have sought to undercut his claims by enumerating the multiple ways in which commons are in fact rationally and sustainably "regulated through communal rules and practices" (Ecologist 1993, 13).[4]

A number of groups have attempted to use the notion of a "global commons" as an organizing principle for treaties and international zones such as the seas and outer space, which exist beyond the jurisdiction of individual nation-states. One of the early success stories of this movement was the decision by the United Nations to declare the international sea beds part of the "common heritage" of all humans, and thus a realm that could not be owned.[5] Yet a certain tension exists between the valorization of local commons and theories of global commons such as the seas. Where the advocates of local commons tend to stress the rights of individual communities against "homogenizing" international laws, advocates of the global commons stress the need for precisely such overarching laws, without which, they contend, the seas will be overgrazed, the atmosphere and Antarctica overpolluted, and space over-cluttered. In addition, the tendency of first world corporations to treat the "wild plants, microbes, and cultural knowledge" as part of a "global commons" from which they can freely draw has encouraged the development of international protocols, such as the U N Convention on Biological Diversity (1992), which effectively designate "resources once . . . characterized as part of the *international* commons . . . as *national* sovereignty" (Hayden 2003, 64).

The terminology of land-based commons was first extended to biomedical products and services in the mid-1970s. Renée Fox and Judith Swazey note that Howard Hiatt's article "Protecting the Medical Commons: Who is Responsible" (1975) reframed discussions of organ transplantation in terms of a "commons" of shared goods and hospital services (Fox and Swazey 1992, 235–41). While the notion of a medical commons of organs and hospital services was intended to stress the *shared* nature of these resources, proponents also used this concept to stress the *limited* nature of these organs and services. Failure to recognize the limited nature of these resources, authors such as Hiatt argued, had encouraged a demand for expensive therapies that had escalated beyond reasonable levels. The result, he contended, was an imminent tragedy of the biomedical commons, as the demand for organs outpaced the supply, and as expensive transplant procedures drew resources away from therapies that could benefit far more people (Hiatt 1975). Thus in its first incarnation, the notion of the biomedical commons was founded on the premise of scarcity, serving primarily to emphasize the very limited nature of body parts and medical services (Fox and Swazey 1992, 73–92).[6]

The foundation for a radically different understanding of the biomedical commons, based on the principles of excess and information, was developed in three arenas in the 1980s: hearings in the U.S. Congress on organ transplantation; the development of conceptions of "biodiversity" in environmentalist and indigenous-rights discourse; and discussions focused on the intersection of computer programming and intellectual property. As we discussed in chapter 3, congressional sponsors of the National Organ Transplantation Act (1984) disputed the claim that organs were a scarce resource, arguing instead that shortages were simply the effects of a lack of information: millions of Americans, they asserted, would be prepared to give their organs if informed of this option, and waste could be minimized through the centralized coordination of matches between organs and recipients.

Principles of information and excess also characterized the various conceptions of biodiversity that were developed in the 1980s and 1990s. Biodiversity first emerged as a key term in environmentalist discourse in the United States as part of an attempt to convince domestic and foreign policymakers that the extinction of animal and plant species was not an economic "externality" capable of being ignored in calculations of corporate and national interests but rather a potentially crippling long-term cost (Hayden 1998; Hayden 2003, 51; Takacs 1996). The biological diversity of the globe was described as a repository of excess—of potential value—that would enable spectacular returns (in terms of both health and financial returns on investment), so long as the multitude of existing plants and animals—and indigenous knowledge of their possible uses—were preserved. Thus for many advocates, "preservation" of biodiversity required treating indigenous groups as "stewards" of nature and local knowledge, and as potential partners or "stakeholders" in efforts to "prospect" promising plants or animals. The transformation of natural biodiversity from potential into actual value also depended upon understanding the "excess" of biodiversity in informational terms, that is, as a "storehouse of information *not yet catalogued*" (Hayden 2003, 57). As Cori Hayden notes, it is the "elasticity and recombinatorial promise of 'information'" "that underwrites the conceptual power and promise of calls for the protection of biodiversity, for advocates suggest that "[u]nlike prospecting for material commodities such as minerals or timber, biodiversity prospecting is not dependent on large-scale harvests of raw materials," but rather focuses on isolating biochemical compounds that can subsequently be synthesized artificially (Hayden 2003, 58).

The link established between information and excess in the biomedical context and in biodiversity discourse resonated with claims by computer "hackers" and intellectual property theorists that "information wants to be free" (Barlow 1994). In the 1980s and 1990s a number of computer programmers and intellectual property scholars began to draw a sharp distinction between information and material products. They maintained that information, unlike tangible goods such as land (or organs), is in essence "non-rivalrous," since many users can possess the "same" copy of a good at the same time. As James Boyle notes, "[i]f I am using the field for grazing, it may interfere with your plans to use it for growing crops. By contrast, a gene sequence, an MP3 file or an image may be used by multiple parties; my use does not interfere with yours" (Boyle 2003, 41). While Boyle focuses on computer-mediated forms of information, his claims are equally applicable to biological tissues such as cell lines that can be copied and distributed without using up the original "source." To describe a good as "information" from this perspective is to make an ontological claim about the potential for multiplication and distribution, irrespective of the relationship of the good to a computer database. Thus in the biomedical context, the distinction between "rivalrous" and "non-rivalrous" goods holds: while organs are a limited and thus rivalrous resource, biomedical "information," whether in the form of genetic sequences or immortal cell lines, is infinitely duplicable. Thus information can never be "overgrazed" in the way that limited goods could be, nor need it be limited to a certain geographical area.

Given this essential excess of information, critics argue that any shortages of informational content—for example, an inability to experiment on a gene sequence because it is patented, or the inability to buy a cell line because it is priced too high—are artificially produced effects of business monopolies which attempt to "enclose" the intrinsic excess of information (Lessig 2001, 238). Critics worry that recent intellectual property legislation and judicial decisions, such as that in *Moore*, constitute precisely such an enclosure. These critics describe three kinds of threat. First, at least in the United States, digitalization can be used to enclose information that is currently in the public domain. While the underlying "facts" in a copyrighted work—for example, the listings in a telephone book—are not protected under copyright law, legislation such as the Uniform Computer Information Transactions Act allows companies to effectively control access to such underlying data by licensing the software used to access the data (Samuelson 2001, 88–89).[7] Second, critics worry that legislation has been used to shuttle "undecided" new forms of data into private hands, rather than make them freely available. For example, the digitalization of genomic data has enabled some groups to patent genes and gene sequences, which then gives them the right to license uses of those genes and sequences as they see fit. Any researcher who experiments on these genes or sequences without negotiating for a license risks a lawsuit for patent infringement. Third, digitalization can prevent material that would have reverted to the public sphere after a certain time from doing so.[8] For critics, all of these measures corrupt and distort the essential nature of information, transforming non-rivalrous goods into rivalrous goods.

Thus the information commons—of which the biomedical commons is a subsection—would be either "a sphere in which contents are free from intellectual property rights" (Samuelson 2001, 82)[9] or a sphere in which intellectual property functions in an effectively nonproprietary fashion. (The latter possibility—that is, the use of intellectual property law to ensure "free access" to information—is exemplified by instruments such as the General Public License, or GPL, which is a form of intellectual property; more on this below.) In the view of advocates of the commons, protection from the exclusivity generally associated with intellectual property claims will ensure that the non-rivalrous nature of information—its capacity for "infinite" duplication and distribution—is not distorted by "artificial" enclosures. As Lawrence Lessig has noted, this is primarily a question of access: an information commons does not necessarily mean that information has zero cost, only that "if there is a cost, it is a neutrally imposed or equally imposed cost" (Lessig 1998, 1788). For many if not most proponents of a biomedical and informational commons, this approach to intellectual property represents a compromise between individual and collective claims. The information commons would not preempt all forms of intellectual property, but it would protect a central core of information from exclusive property claims. Thus organizations such as Open Bioinformatics Forum, Creative Commons, and BIOS have sought to create institutional structures for maintaining such a commons and facilitating the transfer of information between researchers.[10]

This conception of the information commons has much in common with earlier notions of "the public domain," and in fact it is best understood as an attempt to theorize a "positive" version of the public domain. Boyle notes that contemporary understandings of the "public domain" are relatively recent: while criticisms of intellectual property have been common since at least the 1960s, it was only in the early 1980s that the "public domain" became theorized as such (Boyle 2003, 58–63). However, as Litman (1990) and Frow (1997) have noted, the public domain has tended to be a "purely residual" concept: "rather than being itself a set of specific rights, the public domain is that space, that possibility of access, which is left over after all other rights have been defined and distributed" (Frow 1997, 209). The "information commons," by contrast, is an attempt to constitute a "positive" sphere of protection for information, rather than relegate it to the space left over after commodity rights have been acknowledged.[11]

The Moral Slippery Slope, Jurassic Park, and Innovation Extinction: Arguments for the Biomedical Commons In their attempts to critique "enclosures" of the information commons, commentators have developed at least three rationales to explain why we should fear such transgressions. We shall call these the moral slippery slope, the Jurassic Park, and the innovation extinction arguments. All three are grounded in tragic narrative structures: that is, all three propose that enclosing the commons will put fundamental values into conflict with each other, and the result will be the ruin and loss of at least one fundamental value, and perhaps many. However, beyond this structural agreement, advocates of the three rationales differ markedly in the values that they see threatened by the enclosure of biomedical information.

The moral slippery slope argument is grounded in the claim that transforming non-rivalrous biological tissue and information into commodities will lead eventually to property claims over entire human individuals. According to this logic, seemingly benign patents on components of the biomedical commons—for example, patents on genes and gene sequences—will eventually lead to the enslavement of human bodies. One of the justices in the *Moore* case employed this logic, and it has dominated popular critiques of biocommerce. Andrew Kimbrell, for example, describes *Moore* as an "invas[ion] of the body commons," and he concludes his discussion of that case with the image of patents on "genetically altered human bod[ies]" (Kimbrell 1997, 252, 254). The essential value under attack in this rationale is "dignity," which is threatened by lesser values such as wealth and profit. Advocates of the moral slippery slope rationale generally do not oppose biomedical research per se, or the circulation of tissues and biomedical information, but simply attempts to enclose information through intellectual property regimes.

As we noted in chapter 3, the moral slippery slope line of argument is particularly vulnerable to appropriation by legal and corporate authorities, which have developed strategies to explain how dignity, intellectual property, and public health can be harmoniously coordinated. In *Moore*, for example, the majority justices wrote that dignity was best protected by prohibiting individuals from owning their own tissues, while public health was promoted by strengthening an "information ecology" within which universities produced patentable information and tissues, and then leased them to corporations for therapeutic development. The court suggested that the moral slippery slope argument had no necessary connection to the enclosure of the bioinformatics commons, and as a result both dignity and public health could be protected precisely through strong intellectual property rights.

To focus attention more squarely on the relationship between the production of biovalue and the biomedical commons, other critics have developed what we call the Jurassic Park argument. In the novel and movie of that name, commercial developers believe that they can control and contain bioengineered and patented organisms within a for-profit theme park. However, both corporate piracy and nature's own uncontrollable innovation propel these bioengineered organisms outside the control of capitalist development, and threaten the lives of everyone in the park.[12] Critics who adopt the Jurassic Park rationale believe that patents on biological components will lead to situations of extreme biological vulnerability. Jurassic Park critics such as Vandana Shiva (1997) argue that because these patented products have been produced in isolation from the traditional "intellectual commons" of both land and information, the long-term biological viability of these newly patented products is seriously compromised. Shiva employs the notion of a "traditional intellectual commons" to explore the processes of exchange (of biological materials such as seeds and animals, and of knowledge) that occur in "villages among farmers, in forests among tribespeople and even in universities among scientists" (Shiva 1997, 10). While advocates of intellectual property often insist that devices such as patents are necessary to promote innovation, critics such as Shiva contend that there are in fact "diverse traditions of creativity" fostered by the traditional intellectual commons (Shiva 1997, 8), and groups such as the International Society of Ethnobiology, in their Declaration of Belém (1988), contend that "native peoples have been stewards of 99 percent of the world's genetic resources and . . . there is an inextricable link between cultural and biological diversity" (cited in Hayden 2003, 35).

Shiva notes, moreover, the lack of evidence that patents in fact encourage innovation (Shiva 1997, 9–15). She emphasizes that the "innovation" purportedly encouraged by intellectual property regimes— that is, the production of biovalue through the multiplication and distribution of tissues and information—disguises a much more fundamental homogenizing tendency of intellectual property. Corporate biovalue is produced only to the extent that it can be incorporated into globalized and standardized production and distribution patterns. Companies such as Monsanto, for example, engineer and patent plant species in part so that they can sell uniform seeds as well as accompanying fertilizers and pesticides to worldwide markets. Yet such biological uniformity makes engineered organisms particularly vulnerable to "wild" viruses and organisms, with the result that "patents on life enclose the creativity inherent to living systems" (Shiva 1997, 7). Consequently, enclosure of the traditional intellectual biocommons both stifles human innovation and drives natural "innovation" into hyper-development outside corporately controlled systems, into the realm of pathogens and viruses. Thus "[e]cological vulnerability comes from the fact that species and ecosystems have been engineered and controlled to such an extent that they lose the capacity to adapt and evolve" (Shiva 1997, 31). Just as the bioengineered dinosaurs of *Jurassic Park* destroy their bioengineers, enclosure of the bioinformatics commons stunts the capacity for adaptation in selected engineered organisms, inadvertently encouraging the evolution of opportunistic organisms.[13] Where moral slippery slope critics positioned the enclosure of the bioinformatics commons as the first step in a process that would lead to moral destitution, Jurassic Park critics position enclosure as the first step in a process that will lead to greater sickness—and possible extinction—of humans and other animals.

The emphasis on biological disaster associated with the Jurassic Park rationale is not meant to deny the strong element of moral condemnation that has attended this line of argumentation. Shiva, as well as indigenous-rights groups such as the Indigenous Peoples Council on Biocolonialism and the ETC Group (formerly the Rural Advancement Foundation International, or RAFI), repeatedly characterizes the assertion of intellectual property rights as "biopiracy" or "bioprospecting."[14] While these clearly are terms of moral disapprobation, the moral question of adjudicating the rights of source and recipient is in fact a logically secondary question for Jurassic Park critics. The primary rationale is pragmatic, not moral: for Jurassic Park critics, the enclosure of the commons may be morally degrading but much more fundamentally it is biologically dangerous.

Where Jurassic Park critics tend to be drawn from the ranks of indigenous-rights advocacy, a third rationale for the biomedical commons has been developed within the sphere of legal criticism. We call this the innovation extinction argument. The language of "innovation extinction" emerged in the late 1970s in the testimony of witnesses before congressional patent reform committees. As we noted in chapter 3, witnesses arguing for stronger private patent rights contended that the patent regime then current threatened to "extinguish" the creative potential of the nation. For example, Howard I. Forman, deputy assistant secretary of commerce for product standards, contended that the ability of the U.S. government to take title to inventions produced with federal funding amounted to "suppression or extinction of some of our limited reservoir of national assets" (U.S. Congress 1976, 17). While Forman and his allies successfully altered patent legislation, the language of innovation extinction reemerged in the late 1990s, this time employed by advocates of the commons. These innovation extinction critics contend that legislation permitting private ownership of the biomedical commons undercuts its own foundations, because it destroys the capacity for further human innovation. For these critics, human innovation—whether in the form of computer code, genetic research, or therapeutic product development—requires a foundation, or "layer," of basic materials that can be freely mixed and combined, and this foundation or layer is only guaranteed by maintaining a commons of accessible intellectual materials. Jessica Litman, for example, sees an intellectual commons as a necessary "device that permits the rest of the [intellectual property] system to work by leaving the raw material of authorship available for authors to use" (Litman 1990, 968). Since information is a non-rivalrous resource, one cannot predict who will use it, or how users will combine its contents in new and interesting ways. This unpredictable sort of cross-fertilization is precisely the strength of the intellectual commons, and the foundation for innovation. Yet as Lawrence Lessig notes, current intellectual property laws tend to hinder access to the basic layer of information and tissues, and fear of lawsuits deters people from making innovative use of these "raw materials." Critics such as Lessig and Litman fear that where previously a basic layer of ideas and information was left free, recent legislation seeks to commodify this foundation, thus destroying the necessary condition of innovation. Since, they contend, the precondition of human innovation is a free exchange of knowledge and materials, property structures that undercut this gift economy—for example, overly strong intellectual property regimes—threaten to destroy their own foundations.

While innovation extinction critics dispute Hardin's central claim that the commons is an unviable institution, they have nevertheless adopted his basic schema. "Corporations" have taken the place of Hardin's "herdsmen," but the result is the same. If corporations are allowed to enclose the intellectual commons, they will destroy the foundation of future innovation, just as Hardin's herdsmen, if unrestrained, destroyed the foundation for future uses of their commons. Lessig notes that Hardin's original claim about the commons far more accurately describes the relationship of modern capitalism to the intellectual commons than it did the relationship of "herdsmen" to a land-based commons, and he rewrites Hardin's original claim accordingly: "Therein lies the tragedy. Each [firm] is locked into a system that compels [it] to increase [its control] without limit: in a world that is limited. *Ruin is the destination toward which all [firms] rush, each pursuing [its] own best interest in a society that believes in the freedom of the commons. Freedom in a commons brings ruin to all"* (Lessig 2001, 175).

By "freedom in a commons," Lessig means "freedom of private interests to turn the commons into property," and thus he and fellow advocates have supported institutions that would limit the freedom of corporations to "enclose" the intellectual commons. This emphasis on the explicit protection of an intellectual commons also distinguishes these critics from the justices in *Moore*. Both the *Moore* justices and innovation extinction critics agree that donations must be protected, for they underwrite the very existence of intellectual property claims. However, where the *Moore* justices sought to protect these donations in a defensive manner, by denying individuals the right to enclose the intellectual commons, innovation extinction critics have taken a more offensive approach by developing institutions that explicitly code information and tissues as part of the intellectual commons.

In the realm of biology and medicine, open-source initiatives have taken several forms. Groups such as the Open Bioinformatics Foundation, the Bioinformatics Organization, and the SNP Consortium allow free web access to DNA, RNA, protein sequences, and SNP's databases, as well as free access to GPL-licensed software for analyzing the data (which often take the form of biologically oriented versions of open-source software applications—for example BioPerl, BioPython, Bio-XML, BioJava, BioCORBA, BioLisp, BioRuby). In an "open letter to the NIH," J. W. Bizzaro, a member of the board of directors of the Bioinformatics Organization, outlines the impetus behind these efforts, arguing that current copyright laws are destructive of innovation: "As a result of the current publication model, copyright belongs to non-public entities and not to the researcher or funder, thus depriving the latter parties of their ability to disseminate their very own results. This runs contrary to the spirit of innovation and fair market rules by limiting independent scientists in their ability to share their results after publication" (Bizzaro 2004).[15] Attempting to turn the tables on advocates of strong intellectual property rights, Bizzaro contends that the current intellectual property system has become "now largely obsolete." Other open-source bioinformatics initiatives include a recent proposal for "open-source drug discovery" of therapies for tropical diseases. Pharmaceutical companies have been reluctant to focus research on these diseases, since sufferers are often desperately poor and therefore not desirable consumers. The Tropical Disease Initiative

(TDI) seeks to compensate for this lack of interest by linking bio-informatic computation, "wet" lab experiments, and peer review in an informal network, which would (its proponents claim) allow TDI researchers to "discover drug candidates in much the same way that LINUX builds operating systems" (Maurer, Rai, and Sali 2004).

For the most part these critics who advocate open-source solutions are not opposed to intellectual property but see the information commons and intellectual property as bound in a necessary relationship to one another. Legal critics such as Boyle and Lessig contend that if there is a possible tragedy of the information commons, it stems not from the possibility of overgrazing a good (an impossibility in the case of information) but from problems with incentives. That is, why will people create information goods if they can be so easily copied? Why, for example, would a researcher labor to create an immortal cell line from John Moore's diseased spleen if she knew that upon completion, it could be freely distributed to researchers throughout the globe? To address this problem and provide the incentives to produce informational goods, these critics assert that some intellectual property rights must be left intact, but they object to the complete enclosure of the information commons. For these critics the commodity, in the form of intellectual property, is necessary, but its precondition is the gift, in the form of the commons.[16] Critics such as Lessig argue that a judicious combination of intellectual commons and intellectual property actually increases the values associated with property and capitalism: "a commons can have value greater than the same assets would if enclosed" (Lessig 2001, 236). The intellectual commons maintains an originary "outside of property" (Boyle 2003, 62), which allows for the free circulation of ideas and products, but property provides a "supplement," in the form of incentives, that ensures the transformation of these common resources into specific therapeutic products.

Yet like every tale of "supplements," the (primary) origin and (secondary) supplement seem continually to slide into one another. What brings into relief this elision of the difference between the two in the context of the information commons is that many (if not all) the legal tools used to "protect" the commons are in fact intellectual property instruments, such as "open-source" software and databases, the General Public License (GPL), and most modes of the "creative commons" contracts. So, for example, while the General Public License sets out to "guarantee your freedom to share and . . . make sure the software is free for all its users," it achieves this goal within, not outside, the system of intellectual property, since it is, after all, an intellectual property license.[17] Thus the commons that at first appeared to be *outside* of property frequently turns out to be a specific mode of property, rather than its opposite. The emphasis of innovation extinction theorists on the need to protect the commons through intellectual property instruments makes them uneasy allies of Jurassic Park critics, who are generally suspicious of attempts to refigure the commons as a mode of property.

Jurassic Park and innovation extinction critics tend to understand the contours of the biomedical or information commons differently. For innovation extinction critics, the capacity of information for infinite distribution means that the information commons must be global; or, more precisely, not restricted to a particular place. Jurassic Park critics often favor much more local approaches, noting that a globalized commons in fact encourages corporate globalization of local markets. They describe notions such as the "common heritage of mankind" as an extension of colonialism: rather than enabling modes of local control, a globally open biocommons "[t]reats indigenous knowledge and third world biodiversity as open access systems" that can only be protected through intellectual property instruments (Shiva et al. 1997, 6).

The Corporate Protection of the Commons: Affymetrix   Despite these apparent differences, the Jurassic Park and innovation extinction rationales depend on very similar logics. Both seek to outline conditions of innovation, though the Jurassic Park rationale focuses on both human innovation and the natural innovation that is part of the process of evolution, while the innovation extinction rationale focuses solely on human innovation. Both, moreover, suggest that stagnation is the result of enclosure. For innovation extinction theorists such as Boyle and Lessig, this stagnation affects human intellectual developments; for Jurassic Park theorists such as Shiva, stagnation leads to overly protected "garden" organisms and ecosystems, vulnerable to wild viruses. Both suggest that the best defense against the problems of stagnation is a healthy commons—a gift domain outside of property that allows ideas and genetic material to be exchanged freely, back and forth. For innovation extinction critics, protecting intellectual property is only possible if one protects its foundation, the gifts of the commons. For Jurassic Park theorists, protecting public health is only possible if one protects its source, natural biodiversity, and this is possible only because of the free exchange that goes on in the intellectual commons.

Recognizing the appeal of both positions, some corporations have begun to market their products through a clever combination of the two, arguing with Shiva that public health requires a commons of intellectual products, and with Boyle and Lessig that the gifts of the commons should be supplemented by intellectual property. Perhaps the most successful of these corporations is Affymetrix, which sells, among other products, gene chips (DNA microarrays). These products allow researchers to test the expression of a large number of genes at the same time. As Affymetrix stresses on its web site and in its promotional literature, this capability has important implications for such life-threatening diseases as cancer, a claim repeated by medical associations and the news media. For example, the web site provides a link to an article in the *Journal of the American Medical Association* in which Brian Vastag suggests that microarrays such as those produced by Affymetrix "will someday tell clinicians whether a patient's early stage cancer will metastasize, or if it will respond to chemotherapy" (Vastag 2003, 155). Affymetrix's corporate portfolio is based on patents—it holds more than 230 U.S. patents and has 400 more pending—but it has taken a very strong and public position against the patenting of genes and gene sequences, arguing that it is vital to protect a commons of genetic information.[18] The fundamental reason for Affymetrix's resistance to gene and gene sequence patents is fairly clear: its gene chips are attractive because they allow researchers to test the expression of multiple genes all at once; however, if researchers have to obtain separate licenses for each gene that they want to test, the utility of the gene chip will be seriously hindered. Thus while Affymetrix wants a level of patent protection for devices such as the gene chip, it would like to prevent patents on the subject of its testing device (genes). As Barbara Caulfield, legal counsel of Affymetrix, put it, patents are good at the level of "tests, therapeutic proteins, [and] particular methods for approaching a clinical experiment," but should not be allowed at the level of genes.[19]

While representatives of Affymetrix are willing to acknowledge this self-interested logic, they have chosen to cast their claims in more general, theoretical terms, and have developed an interesting combination of the Jurassic Park and innovation extinction rationales outlined above. Affymetrix argues that its dilemma—that is, the desire to keep patents at one level but forbid them at a more "primary" level—is not unique, and will come to characterize many testing companies and concerns. As a result, Affymetrix contends that there must be a biomedical commons upon which future testing devices and therapies can be developed. Like Boyle and Lessig, it does not see the commons as a hindrance to commerce or patents but as its enabling condition; without the free exchange of information, and free access to genes and gene sequences, there can be no commodities such as the gene chip. However, Affymetrix also supplements this "invention" logic with fears drawn from the Jurassic Park line of argumentation, stressing that its products will help accurately diagnose life-threatening diseases such as cancer. Affymetrix puts an especial stress on cancer, a disease which—as an example of natural innovation "gone wild"— subtly helps to reinforce the message that Affymetrix's products will control, not contribute to, deadly natural innovation. (And as a corollary, this line of reasoning suggests that gene patents, since they hinder use of the gene chip, are vectors of the further spread of disease.) Moreover, Affymetrix stresses that its chips will enable personalized predictions of drug efficacy, thereby hinting that it too is working against the sort of biological "standardization" that eco-activists such as Shiva fear. For Affymetrix, as for Shiva, the gifts of the intellectual commons are the foundation of biological viability itself.

Affymetrix's position depends on the implicit premise that a biomedical commons will enable the harmonious coordination of natural and human modes of "innovation." This was precisely the position outlined in the Bayh-Dole Act, and reaffirmed by the majority in the *Moore* decision: both suggested that public health depended upon the production of biovalue within an information ecology of research "donations" and corporate property. Affymetrix grafts the institution of the bioinformatics commons to this logic. The authors of "The Genetic Age: Who Owns the Genome?" contend: "Policymakers face the daunting task of constructing, interpreting and administering a framework of laws and regulations that must strike a balance between the private sector's need to reward innovation and the public's right to reap the benefits and advances in genomics in order to improve the quality of our lives" (Brown et al. 2002, 8). Affymetrix argues that policymakers can accomplish this daunting task by establishing a biomedical commons. While both the Jurassic Park and invention theorists would probably see Affymetrix's combination of these "logics of the commons" as an example of self-interested opportunism, Affymetrix's support of the commons makes it difficult to know how one could consistently distinguish "good" from "bad" uses of the commons. The essence of both the Jurassic Park and innovation extinction arguments is that the gift is the enabling condition of biodiversity and biovalue, and Affymetrix has taken precisely the same position, seeking to protect a layer of genetic information that it claims will enable therapeutic innovation.

PXE International and the Communities of the Commodity   Even as Affymetrix has initiated a corporate appropriation of the language of the gift, at least one patient rights group has begun to work in the opposite direction by asserting the primacy of the commodity. PXE International is a nonprofit corporation established by Patrick and Sharon Terry, whose children suffer from pseudoxanthoma elasticum (PXE), a rare, progressive disease that causes premature aging of cells (with symptoms such as vision impairment, skin lesions, and an extremely abridged life span).[20] The Terrys first approached pharmaceutical companies as supplicants, asking "big pharma" to develop life-extending therapies for their children. However, after receiving little response from the pharmaceutical industry (which in general is reluctant to develop therapies for diseases that afflict only a small population), the Terrys took two radical measures. First, in cooperation with researchers at the University of Hawaii, they were able to isolate, and then patent, the gene that causes pseudoxanthoma elasticum. Second, they established a nonprofit corporation responsible for licensing use of this gene to interested researchers, and created institutions and protocols that allow PXE International to direct its own international flows of tissues and information related to this disease. For example, they have created a worldwide network of fifty-six support offices, their own blood and tissue banks, and epidemiological and MRI databanks. Rather than rely on the largesse of the families of those afflicted (as patient groups often do to raise funds), the Terrys have appropriated the commodity form (in this case a patented gene) to create new flows of body tissues and information. In public discussions of their model, they stress that these new flows of tissues and information are patient-oriented (not doctor- or corporation-oriented), in that they seek to create a worldwide patient rights community, within which data and therapies will circulate freely. What they seek to create, in short, is a patient commons (at least for those patients afflicted with PXE). While this patient commons depends upon U.S. patent law (and its global extension through reciprocal trade agreements), it situates these national allegiances within a set of diversified forms of global belonging and obligation, as described by Urry (2000).

The Terrys stress that the origin and basis of this commons is the commodity, in the form of the PXE patent (as well as related commodities, such as the contents of PXE biobanks and the information generated from clinical trials). Sharon Terry, "co-inventor" (along with the University of Hawaii) of the PXE gene and president of Genetic Alliance, asserts that PXE International "use[s] a commodity to: (a) create a community; (b) leverage funding; [and] (c) coordinate the research" associated with therapies and a possible cure for the disease.[21] The PXE patent enables this research community in part because it has allowed PXE International to have access to venture capital in ways that were not otherwise possible. While pharmaceutical companies remain uninterested in a disease that afflicts relatively few people, they are well aware that the pseudoxanthoma elasticum gene may play a partial role in other, more lucrative, diseases, and they will need to negotiate with PXE International to gain access to the PXE gene. Patrick Terry argues that PXE International deploys its patent in ways that encourage research on PXE, and thus facilitates the interests of patients and their families, not corporations. Terry contends that this approach allows patient rights groups to move away from the "trickle-down" model of benefits—in which corporations promise benefits only in the form of drugs and therapies that will appear "sometime" in the future—and toward a model in which patient groups are given support in various ways throughout the research process. By using its patent as a "lure," and in cooperation with related patient-rights organizations such as International Genetic Alliance, PXE has established partnerships with corporations such as Affymetrix, Incyte Inc., and Genomic Health (a new company which shares co-founders with Incyte Inc. and Genentech).

The Terrys also contend that through licensing, the patent gives them continuing flexibility. Patents award "ownership" over a gene or gene sequence, but the ownership right can be sold, or assigned, by means of license rights which can be structured in a variety of ways, leaving the lessee with rights ranging from free access to very limited access. PXE International is willing to license use of the gene under a number of different conditions: for example, free use for researchers working on therapies for pseudoxanthoma elasticum, and profit-sharing agreements for corporations not interested in those sorts of therapies. Thus, according to the Terrys, the commodity not only enables (and is thus logically prior to) the formation of the "gift" research community of PXE patients, but also allows this community to grow and adapt.

While PXE International has encouraged the creation of international alliances and tissue exchanges, it does not aim to create a unitary, global biomedical commons, nor does it seek to create "local" commons that are delimited within national spaces. Rather, in its model commons emerge around particular problems, tissues, or informational nodes (for PXE International itself, the PXE disease and gene). On the one hand, this approach seems to privilege a neoliberal model of competing groups of "stakeholders," who circulate tissues and information within their groups but jealously guard against "free" dissemination to outsiders. Moreover, it threatens to tie research and the structures through which information circulates to current understandings of disease entities. On the other hand, though, this approach has enabled a mode of gathering and circulating tissue and information that does not treat people as resources to be "mined" but instead includes them within the informational flows normally accessible only to researchers and corporations. This understanding of

commodities is reminiscent of the description by Douglas and Isherwood of commodity flows as "live information systems," in which
commodities are "both the hardware and the software, so to speak, of
an information system whose principal concern is to monitor its own
performance" (Douglas and Isherwood 1979, xiv, 49). They suggest
that different information systems of commodity exchange can be
assessed morally according to their degree of inclusiveness: that is, do
systems of commodity exchange hinder or facilitate ever more inclusive interpersonal interactions? From this perspective, PXE International has attempted to employ the commodity as a device that will
include, as agents, a greater number of people in flows of tissue and
information.

Innovation, Gifts, and Commodities Affymetrix and PXE International thus represent two opposing claims concerning the relationship
between the bioinformatics commons, research, and community values. Affymetrix claims that a global information commons is the necessary foundation for both research and health-related commodities,
while PXE International claims that a commodity is the necessary
condition of local research commons and eventual therapies. However, rather than attempt to determine which of these two perspectives
is "correct," it is more useful to read this conflict of interpretations as
highlighting the specific ways in which the categories of the commons
and the commodity are dependent on each other (for example, Affymetrix and PXE International are cosponsors of the nonprofit group
Genetic Alliance). Moreover, notwithstanding the conflict over the relative priorities of gifts and commodities, "innovation" is the common
ground of this argument: even as they dispute the nature of the ecology that supports innovation, all parties involved agree that it is a
fundamental value.

Recent anthropological and sociological theory on the gift-commodity
distinction has stressed the extent to which these two categories are
entwined, and this analysis applies to the concept of the biomedical
commons as well. In the view of Frow (1997), we should understand
this entwinement of gift and commodity as both logical and historical.
Their logical entwinement—that is, the impossibility of defining the
essence of one category without making recourse to properties that

supposedly are found only in the other—has been the focus of deconstructive criticism of the gift (Derrida 1992; Gasché 1997). However, sociological and anthropological critics such as Bourdieu (1977), Weiner (1992), Strathern (1988), and Frow (1997) have outlined historical entwinements of the categories of gift and commodity, most frequently through empirical studies; according to these authors, gift giving, in particular contexts and for particular groups, in fact embodies the same "forms of calculation, strategy, and motivation" that supposedly define commodity exchange. The point of such logical or historical deconstructions of the gift-commodity distinction is not to render these categories useless but to reveal that they are poles within a system, not autonomous, competing systems. Critics interested in the logical entwinement of these categories focus on the concepts and premises that allow these to appear as separate systems, while critics interested in historical entwinement investigate the rituals, practices, and institutions that perpetuate the illusion of separate spheres.

Affymetrix exemplifies the "corporate" logic of the biomedical commons, while PXE International exemplifies the assumptions that have allowed the biomedical commons to appear separate from commodities while also serving as the ground for commodities. Most descriptions of the bioinformatics commons draw heavily on the rhetoric of the gift, portraying the commons as a realm in which gift relations dominate. For Jurassic Park critics such as Shiva, for example, the traditional intellectual commons is the site of *gyan daan*, or the "gifting" of agricultural materials such as seeds (Shiva 1997, 68, 122). For innovation extinction theorists such as Boyle and Lessig—and for corporations such as Affymetrix—the ability to freely appropriate the intellectual materials of the information commons enables all intellectual property claims. Just as John Locke's land-based commons was "always already" there before its enclosure, so too do both Jurassic Park and innovation extinction critics position the biomedical commons as a space that logically preexists its enclosure, even if in actual fact its informational "contents" are being created in the present. The example of Affymetrix demonstrates how these understandings of the commons are tied to specific assumptions about property, the global circulation of information, and hopes for medical therapies. Yet as the founders of PXE International stress, versions of the biomedical com-

mons do not emerge *ex nihilo*, and then wait to be enclosed or protected, but are always already human creations, and to bring them into
existence requires resources and organization. One need not accept
the Terrys' implicit naturalization of the neoliberal "stakeholder" to
recognize with them that the model of the information commons as
simply "out there" and self-propagating ignores how concrete social
processes allow information to be generated and distributed. Even
more strikingly, PXE International achieves precisely the goal of Jurassic Park critics—that is, localized rather than globalized commons—
yet it accomplishes this through the instrument (intellectual property)
viewed with so much suspicion by these critics. In doing so, however,
PXE International transforms the meaning of both "the local" (not
necessarily tied to a particular place, but rather to particular configurations of bodies) and "the global" (denoting exchanges across national
lines, but without necessarily aspiring to cosmopolitanism).

The logical and historical entwinement of gifts and commodities in
current discussions of the biomedical commons are knotted together
through the concept of innovation. For innovation extinction theorists
such as Boyle and Lessig, the fundamental need for innovation means
that the commons cannot be imagined without intellectual property,
because in the absence of intellectual property there would be few
incentives to innovate and the information commons would lie fallow.
Jurassic Park critics such as Shiva are far less committed to the principle that innovation depends upon property, but equally committed to
the value of innovation (both human and natural). Shiva's rejection of
property as a requirement for innovation depends upon what sometimes appears to be a naïve reliance on problematic notions of "primitive gifts" between nonwestern groups, and it is questionable whether
her representation of distributed systems of "local" regimes of innovation differs markedly from the ideology (if not the reality) of neoliberal
capitalist competition between different firms.[22]

Gift and commodity have become confused in discussions of the
biomedical commons because the gift and the commons have been
called upon to perform the function traditionally aligned with commodities and capitalist production: the production of biovalue. Waldby
has suggested that "biovalue is generated wherever the generative and
transformative productivity of living entities can be instrumentalized

along lines that make them useful for human projects—science, industry, medicine, agriculture or other arenas of technical culture" (Waldby 2000, 33). Critics have generally tied the production of biovalue to the system and economies of late capitalist commodity production, but proponents of the biocommons have, intentionally or not, rewritten the commons as a site of biovaluable production. Frow provides a useful summary of the "powers" frequently attributed to the system of commodity production, noting that the commodity form is generally understood to "d[o] three things": "First, it channels resources of capital into an area of production in order to expand it to its fullest capacity, at the same time destroying all productive aspects which are not themselves commodified. Second, it transforms the purpose of production away from the particular qualities of the thing produced and towards the generation of profit . . . Third, it transforms previously or potentially common resources . . . into private resources" (Frow 1997, 138). Both Jurassic Park and innovation extinction critics are solidly critical of Frow's third function of commodities (enclosure of the commons), and respectively more and less suspicious of the value of profit. However, both camps agree that the production of biovalue is either the fundamental value (Jurassic Park) or one of several fundamental values (innovation extinction). Jurassic Park critics contest claims that systems of capitalist commodity production can fully develop biovalue, contending instead that the traditional intellectual commons provides the most effective means of maximizing biovalue. Innovation extinction critics also contest the claim that intellectual property instruments, on their own, can produce biovalue; they contend that the production of biovalue requires a commons.

6

Real-Time Demand

INFORMATION, REGENERATION,

AND ORGAN MARKETS

In the opening scenes of Stephen Frears's film *Dirty Pretty Things* (2002), Okwe (Chiwetel Ejiofor), a former Nigerian doctor now working illegally in London as a hotel clerk, discovers a human heart clogging the toilet in one of the suites. As the film unfolds, Okwe discovers that his employers are at the center of an international for-profit organ transplantation ring that forces illegal immigrants in London to sell their kidneys or other "spare" body parts for cash and passports. The film ends on an upbeat note. Okwe and his Turkish friend Senay (Audrey Tautou) obtain passports and escape from Britain—Okwe to Nigeria and Senay to the United States—without having to participate in this illicit organ economy. Moreover, they are able to turn the tables on one of the organ marketeers, using Okwe's medical knowledge to drug and incapacitate him. While the beginning of the film literalizes the fear that human values associated with the heart, such as dignity and compassion, are being overwhelmed by the cannibal forces of late capitalism, dignity and individual agency prevail in the end. Okwe's and Senay's escape from the global organ trade thus lends itself to an allegorical reading, suggesting that late capitalism contains the seeds of its own destruction. Even as it encourages the global diaspora of illegal workers such as Okwe and Senay, by that same logic it enables these workers to disrupt the system in its global centers.

Frears's film appeared in the same year as a well-publicized scandal of two British physicians who had agreed to help undercover journalists obtain organs from live donors in India.[1] The journalists' eyewitness account brought to public attention a series of illegal organ transplantation networks that spanned the globe. Since the early 1980s "fringe" human rights groups had sought to convince the broader public of such markets, but it was these later events, and others like it, that brought reports to the front page of broadsheet newspapers like the *New York Times*. Prosecutors and journalists outlined the activities of illegal organ marketeers who connect wealthy individuals in developed countries such as the United Kingdom, the United States, and Israel with desperately poor people willing to sell organs (primarily kidneys) in countries such as Turkey, Brazil, and Iraq. While Frears's film collapses the global dimension of these markets into the confines of London, journalistic and academic accounts have outlined complicated networks that often require airplane flights between several countries for both the sellers and the buyers of kidneys (Hughes 1991; Scheper-Hughes 2000; Finkel 2001). Frears's film also highlights the increasing tension between two economies of organ transfer. On the one hand we find state-regulated organ donation systems that are supposed to govern the demand for organ transplantation in countries such as the United Kingdom and the United States; on the other, an apparently increasing number of illegal organ "markets" allow the relatively wealthy to find organs more quickly than is possible within the legal transplantation system. This tension has encouraged an increasing number of lawyers, economists, and bioethicists to advocate for the creation of legal organ markets, a development that would, these proponents contend, both make legal organ transplantation more efficient and equitable and end the demand driving the black markets in organs.

This chapter outlines the history of organ transplantation in the United States, focusing especially on this increasing interest in legalized markets to mediate organ exchange. While the nature, efficiency, and morality of such markets have been the subject of an extraordinary number of legal, economic, sociological, anthropological, and bioethical articles and monographs, this chapter focuses on connections between organ transplantation and the tissue economies outlined in previous chapters. We contend that contemporary discussions of organ transplantation—and especially discussions of the need for more efficient and productive organ markets—must be understood in the context of the speculative tissue economies outlined in our chapters on cord blood, stem cells, and cell lines.[2] These economies, as we have seen, promise to deliver self-regenerating bodies at some time in the future, but so far have produced very few clinical therapies.[3] We suggest in this chapter that the spectacular investment of venture capital and research and development funds into regenerative therapies, tissues, and medicines has fueled expectations about the imminent arrival of these life-extending technologies, and created a cultural desire for, and sense of entitlement to, self-regeneration among the aging populations of the wealthy North. This in turn has put tremendous pressure on "real-time" therapies such as organ transplantation, which like blood donation rely on the regenerative capacities of another's body. In the United States the "national body" of organ-donating fellow citizens has not proved capable of supplying an organ surplus able to meet demand. This shortfall has led to a search in other sites and through market rather than gift economies. So "spare" kidneys in third world bodies are resignified as a negotiable surplus, and more and more analysts and commentators in the United States, the United Kingdom, and elsewhere call for the establishment of national, regulated markets in organs.

We begin by outlining the history of organ transplantation debates in the United States, noting that in a series of congressional hearings in the early 1980s, organ transplantation was understood as an "information problem," in two senses. First, according to many witnesses successful organ transplantation required the creation of large, computer-mediated information systems that would allow donors and recipients to be quickly matched. In addition, many witnesses testified that the donation system of organ exchange was capable of coordinating the "supply" of, and "demand" for, organs if only information about this form of gift exchange were better disseminated. However, as we outline in this chapter, the promise of the donation system has failed to emerge. The demand for organs in the United States has constantly outstripped the donated supply. Consequently, a number of commentators have seized on the language of supply and demand to argue that a "market" in organs would coordinate information far more effectively (and morally) than a donation system. However, we note that their analyses do not take into account the inflation of expectations and demand both inherent in organ transplant medicine (the expansion and improvement of transplant techniques, for example) and resulting from regenerative biotechnology's claims. We then discuss an attempted auction of a kidney on the commercial site eBay, and argue that this event, whether real or a "hoax," was a symbol, staged within the paradigmatic exemplar of a real-time market, for this conflict between the speculative promise of life-extending technologies and real-time life-extending technologies such as organ transplantation. We conclude with a brief discussion of the links between organ markets and what Cori Hayden calls the "idiom of expectation" typical of contemporary capitalism (Hayden 2003, 65).

The National Organ Transplantation Act: Organ Distribution as an Information Problem   While blood and organs are different kinds of tissues which require very different technologies of transfusion and transplantation, both have been understood as presenting information problems in the United States, and both have been tightly linked to the gift form of exchange. As we discussed in chapter 1, blood donation was understood as an information problem in the 1950s and 1960s in the United States. To begin with, the antitrust charges brought against several Kansas City nonprofit community blood centers were based on the claim that physicians were "conspiring" if they even casually discussed the levels and nature of inter-institutional blood supplies with each other. Many congressional witnesses for the nonprofit agencies countered that the technicity of blood, its short shelf life, and other considerations demanded measures to increase the amount of information shared by physicians, blood banks, and hospitals. This was a debate, in other words, about which kind of system was best able to react to, and minimize, forms of tissue waste. Was the market system best able to perform this function, or was a gift system (connected to a "command economy" of governmental agencies and hospitals) more sensitized to the sites and forms of waste? In the 1960s the unambiguous answer, at least for blood, was that the gift system was far better at monitoring and minimizing waste than the market was.

Organ transplants in the United States were understood within this same paradigm that linked questions of information and waste. Organ transplantation was the focus of public legislation in the United States at two moments: when the Uniform Anatomical Gift Act was enacted in 1968, and again in a series of congressional hearings in the early 1980s. These hearings resulted in the National Organ Transplantation Act of 1984 (and a revised Uniform Anatomical Gift Act in 1987).[4] The increasing survival rates of transplant recipients in the 1960s encouraged state and federal legislators and advisors to consider measures that would increase the number of organ donors, and the Uniform Anatomical Gift Act of 1968 represented an attempt to establish a standard definition of tissue "gifts" that would apply across all states.[5] The consensus at the time was that such a standardization of state laws would remind members of the public of their ability to become donors (thus increasing the supply of organs) and decrease physicians' fears of legal liability when they considered using cadaveric organs (thus decreasing waste).[6]

The development in the late 1970s and early 1980s of better transplantation techniques and more effective immunosuppression drugs (such as cyclosporine A and FK-506) enabled even more widespread transplantation of an expanding array of tissues (kidneys, corneas, hearts, heart-lung combinations, and so on). However, the increased ability to transplant organs also exacerbated the problematic relationship between the "supply" of tissues and the apparently always greater "demand." In addition, the increasing ability to transplant organs and tissues was not always accompanied by an increased willingness on the part of insurance companies to pay for the procedures. These tensions were evident at the national level in July 1983, when President Ronald Reagan made a national radio appeal for a child named Ashley Bailey, who was awaiting a liver transplant. Reagan pleaded for a donor to come forward, and committed the presidential airplane (Air Force One) to transport the organ. Legislators had already begun to debate these same problems, and the president's appeal simply brought increased attention to the need for a national policy; as the chairman of a congressional hearing noted, "Air Force I isn't a national policy" (U.S. Congress 1984a, 3). After a series of lengthy and heavily publicized hearings, Congress passed the National Organ Transplant Act, which among several other provisions explicitly forbade interstate organ sales. It also established a task force to determine the most effective methods for attacking the supply side of the problem, and coordinating the movement of tissues on the demand side (U.S. Task Force on Organ Transplantation 1986, 2, 30).

As we noted in chapter 3, deficits in organ supply were attributed to impeded information flows. Representative Henry Waxman, chairman of the committee holding the hearings, and Representative Al Gore Jr. defended the gift system as fully capable of matching organ supply and demand: Waxman, for example, claimed that 75 percent of Americans would "donate if given the chance" (U.S. Congress 1984a, 287). Both Waxman and Gore ascribed the organ shortages already evident in the early 1980s to the citizenry's lack of knowledge about organ donation. Both also asserted that organ "waste" could be minimized, if not eliminated, by establishing a centralized computer network that would determine appropriate matches between organs and recipients.

However, as one might expect in the era of Reaganomics, it was difficult to cast the problems of organ transplantation in terms of "supply" and "demand" without evoking "the market." In fact, "the market" dominated these discussions of organ transplantation, in two ways. First, though almost all the witnesses at the hearings agreed that some sort of centralized and rationalized network was necessary, there was a disagreement about whether this effort should be initiated by the government or the private, corporate sphere. Dr. Edward Brandt, an assistant secretary for health and Reagan administration witness, testified in favor of letting "the private organizations [establish a national network] themselves" (U.S. Congress 1984a, 176). Another witness sketched out for his listeners a picture of telecommunications companies donating beepers to people on organ waiting lists, and oil companies offering free flights to transport organs (U.S. Congress 1984b, 44). By contrast, the sponsors of the bill—as well as an overwhelming number of the witnesses—favored an organ information network created by the government. Several witnesses pointed out that the government already played a substantial role, through insurance plans such as Medicaid and Medicare, as well as grants, pumping (in Gore's estimation) at least $30 million a year through the current, fragmented system of private networks (U.S. Congress 1984a, 176). Both sides agreed that the fundamental question was one of "efficiency." The administration claimed that a government-sponsored database and network would duplicate the efforts of private companies who would soon step forward to work all this out, while the sponsors claimed that the government could consolidate fragmented private efforts. As a result, both sides found themselves debating the issue in terms of the *values* of the market (efficiency and reduction of waste), even though they disagreed about the precise way to best stimulate the organ economy.

The topic of "the market" also emerged in connection with the possibility of actually selling organs. The creation of an organ market was explicitly proposed by Dr. Barry Jacobs, medical director of the International Kidney Exchange. Jacobs suggested that "[a] fancier computer is not going to solve the problem" of organ shortages and that only the market would coordinate supply and demand. As Gore acknowledged, "[t]he notion [of an organ market] has perhaps a superficial attraction to some because we have all learned that the market system will solve lots of problems if we just stand out of the way and let it work" (U.S. Congress 1984a, 128).

Gore as well as many other witnesses invoked the rhetoric of dignity in an attempt to ward off this threat. Gore contended that a market in organs would result in "dehumanizing people," and he echoed Titmuss's claims about blood sales, hinting that such a market might well lead back to slavery. Chairman Waxman warned his listeners of the "specter of individuals coerced to sell their kidneys" (U.S. Congress 1984a, 125). "It is offensive to make a person's body into a 'thing' for purposes of gain," wrote Dr. Bernard Towers in his testimony for the hearing, making explicit the Kantian logic of these claims. At stake, many witnesses implied, was not simply the fate of the organ donation system in the United States but the very possibility of making "humanity more human," as Waxman put it (U.S. Congress 1984a, 301).

Making humanity more human required liberating several sorts of information flows (and consequently rationalizing the millions of dollars spent by the government on insurance), but it also required a regimen of purity, in which individuals kept their distance from the pollutions of the market. The report of the congressional task force mandated by the act was even more explicit about the dangers of losing collective dignity: the authors of the report "condemn[ed] commercialization of organ transplantation," on the grounds that organs were "a national resource to be used for the public good" and that only a "voluntary donation of organs and tissues by the public" could protect the "dignity of the body" (U.S. Task Force on Organ Transplantation 1986, 9, 15, 29). The authors of the report suggested that commercialization of organ exchange threatened to turn people into means, rather than ends in themselves.

The congressional focus on the relationship between organ transfers, information systems, waste, and the market was formalized in the several years following the congressional hearings. The National Transplantation Act (Public Law 98-507), enacted in 1984, made criminal any attempt to "receive, or otherwise transfer any human organ for valuable consideration for use in human transplantation if the transfer affects interstate commerce."[7] In 1987 the revised Uniform Anatomical Gift Act, a "model act" drafted for consideration by the state legislatures, made it a felony to pay for an organ for the purposes of transplantation in any state, whether or not the transfer affected interstate commerce; like its predecessor the UAGA of 1968, it was adopted by all fifty states. In 1984 the United Network for Organ Sharing (UNOS), a computerized organ information system originally created in 1977 as part of the Southeast Organ Procurement Foundation (SEOPF), became an independent nonprofit entity. In 1986 it was awarded the federal contract to oversee the national Organ Procurement and Transplantation Network (OPTN).

Yet amid this consensus that more efficient flows of information and organs were best facilitated by organ donation rather than a market system, a few commentators acknowledged that the "gift" system worked only to the extent that it was embedded within a market system of health care consumerism. The authors of the task force report, for example, acknowledged that individuals intending to receive a donated organ might very well attempt to select the "best" transplant center based on market competition principles (U.S. Task Force on Organ Transplantation 1986, 112). In addition, hospitals and physicians that performed transplants profited from them, charging insurance companies, Medicare, or Medicaid thousands of dollars to perform operations and monitor their patients' health; the nonprofit organizations that coordinate donor and recipient matches also often collected tens of thousands of dollars for "acquisition charges."[8] As a result, economists such as Barnett and his colleagues have argued, hospitals currently without transplant centers have an interest in establishing one to capture a profitable segment of the health care market (Barnett, Beard, and Kaserman 1993). This asymmetrical logic—that donors should not understand themselves as market players, but both recipients of organs and transplantation providers may, and perhaps must do so—underscores the uneasy relationship between gift and commodity systems of exchange that obtained in these early discussions of organ transplantation.

Organ Markets Reconsidered   In 1983 Dr. Jacobs's argument for creating an organ market was met with derision, but in the two decades since, his proposal has been echoed with increasing frequency. As Donald Joralemon noted in 2001, the "vehement rejection on ethical grounds of anything but uncompensated donation—once the professional norm—has slowly been replaced by an open debate of plans that offer financial rewards to persons willing to have their organs, or the organs of deceased kin, taken for transplantation" (Joralemon 2001, 30). Since the mid-1980s a rather bewildering array of organ market models has been developed, with proposals ranging from an absolutely unregulated market for live organs to a tightly regulated "futures" markets for cadaveric organs. These proposals can be parsed along four basic axes: the source of the organ (cadavers or the living?); the time of payment (present or future?); the "location" of the market (supply side, demand side, or both?); and the mediating agencies (will government and nonprofit agencies facilitate sales and distribution, or will these be handled by for-profit hospitals, private organ brokers, and insurance agencies?).

The vast majority of organ market proposals focus on cadaveric rather than live donations. Many of the proposals for organ markets that were developed in the late 1980s and early 1990s have taken the form of "futures" markets in which an individual agrees to the "harvesting" of organs after his or her death, with payment to go to family members (often in the form of subsidized funeral expenses). Schwindt and Vining first proposed an organ "futures" market in 1986, and the lawyer and economist Lloyd Cohen outlined a very detailed model of such a market in 1989 (Schwindt and Vining 1986; Cohen 1989). The proposal has received increasing support in recent years: in 1995 the Council on Ethical and Judicial Affairs of the American Medical Association seconded the idea of a futures market in cadaver organs, and in 1999 the state of Pennsylvania briefly sought to put into practice a three-year pilot project that offered a $300 funeral expense stipend for families of organ "donors" (Joralemon 2001, 31; see also Joralemon 2000, 224–37). To use terms that we developed in chapter 2, this is an organ market proposal that honors the entangled status of organs. It recognizes their locatedness in networks of family relationships and affects, by directing a small payment not to the organ "owner" but to the bereaved.

A more radical, and less entangled, model of cadaveric organ markets has been advanced by a group of economists led by A. F. Adams, A. H. Barnett, and David L. Kaserman. They have argued for a "spot market," in which organ sellers are compensated in the present for organs to be harvested upon their death, with organ distribution still handled by government or nonprofit agencies (Blair and Kaserman 1991; Barnett, Beard, and Kaserman 1993; Barnett and Kaserman 1995; Adams, Barnett, and Kaserman 1999; Anderson and Barnett 1999; Barnett and Kaserman 2000).[9] This proposal is far less committed to the entangled status of organs than the futures market outlined above, since it treats organ "vendors" as self-subsistent individuals who should be allowed to use their payment in whatever way they wish.

A much smaller number of advocates have proposed "live donor" markets. Most plans focus on kidneys, the easiest organ to donate "live," though some have hinted at the possibility of lung and liver lobe sales. These proposals generally restrict sales to the supply side, with government or nonprofit agencies regulating distribution. In the early 1990s, for example, the British bioethicist John Harris and the philosopher Charles Erin advocated the creation of a government monopsony, in which a government agency would be the sole legal buyer of organs and would control the distribution of kidneys to recipients (Erin and Harris 1994). This plan, Harris and Erin claimed, would "prevent the rich using their purchasing power to exploit the market at the expense of the poor," especially if the organ marketplace was confined "to a particular nation state" or a "regional bloc of states" (Harris and Erin 2002, 114, 115). In 1998 a group of physicians published an article in the *Lancet* that urged readers to reconsider even less restrictive modes of kidney sales. While the authors stressed that they were not proposing an "unfettered market" in kidneys, they sought to prove that arguments against organ sales were in general uncompelling, and concluded with the suggestion "the trade should be regulated rather than banned altogether" (Radcliffe-Richards et al. 1998, 1951).[10]

Whatever the specific plan, proponents of market solutions almost invariably argue that commerce in organs will allow for more efficient and equitable distribution of this "resource." As Joralemon notes, "[v]irtually every article arguing in favor of financial incentives begins with a ritual recitation of the statistics of waiting list deaths" (Joralemon 2001, 33), a rhetorical move designed to highlight the inefficiency of current donation systems. These statistics are certainly impressive: in 1988, for example, 14,742 people in the United States were on organ transplantation waiting lists; the number rose to 33,014 in 1993, 62,415 in 1998, and 87,155 in 2004.[11] The number of people who have died while on organ transplant waiting lists is also sobering: 2,959 in 1993, 5,164 in 1998, and 6,385 in 2002.[12] For market advocates these statistics prove that the donation system is intrinsically incapable of matching supply and demand, and thus financial incentives are needed to "call forth" further supply. Adams, Barnett, and Kaserman have deployed quasi-quantitative supply-and-demand equations and charts to argue that present-time compensation to "donors" for their cadaveric organs would match supply with demand, and at relatively little cost (Barnett, Beard, and Kaserman 1993; Adams, Barnett, and Kaserman 1999). They estimate that a payment of $1,000 to each person for all the organs in his or her cadaver would produce a sufficient organ supply to match demand. Moreover, they claim, such a payment would be far more equitable than the current donation system, which allows

physicians and hospitals to charge insurance companies for operations and follow-up, but denies the donors any access to this money
(Barnett, Beard, and Kaserman 1993). They also point to how the
current donation system encourages the "inefficient" entry of hospitals
into the already saturated transplant market, as each hospital hopes to
capture at least a small number of lucrative transplantation procedures
(Barnett and Kaserman 1995). Thus, while these economists often
claim to leave aside ethical questions when analyzing the comparative
efficiencies of donation and market systems, they clearly believe that
the purportedly greater efficiency of markets is the only ethical solution
to the fact of waiting lists (a conclusion emphasized by the presence of
an epigraph from Ayn Rand—"Every major horror of history was committed in the name of an altruistic motive"—in Barnett and Kaserman
1995, 669).

Proponents of organ markets also argue that regulated financial
compensation for donors would bring under legal control the currently unregulated global black market in organ sales, particularly
kidneys. The history of these black markets is murky, but they seem to
have emerged sometime in the mid-1980s, as a consequence of two
factors. First, the development of immunosuppressant drugs such as
cyclosporine (and later FK-506) reduced the importance of histo-
compatibility. Organs became more standardized and less entangled
in the qualitative specificity of donors and recipients, so that surgeons
could treat them as interchangeable parts rather than as recalcitrant
objects with nearly unique histio-profiles. Such transformations rendered them more compatible with anonymized, market forms of circulation. As Lawrence Cohen notes, "[c]yclosporine *globalizes*, creating
myriad biopolitical fields where donor populations are differentially
and flexibly materialized. Difference is actively suppressed, allowing
specific subpopulations to become 'same enough' for their members
to be surgically disaggregated and their parts reincorporated" (Cohen
2002, 12). Second, illegal markets in organs arguably developed in
response to national legislation that outlawed legal organ markets in
most first world countries. The precise nature of the globalized organ
markets that emerged has been difficult to determine. Many academic
accounts have depended on journalistic sources, such as articles in the
Guardian and the *New York Times* (Bowcott 1989; Bowcott 1990a;

Bowcott 1990b; Parry 1990a; Parry 1990b; Parry 1990c; Parry 1990d; Hughes 1991; Finkel 2001; Allison 2002). These accounts—as well as several well-publicized accounts of organ brokers in the United Kingdom and Brazil—describe international circuits that link various organ recipients and surgeons from developed countries with organ "vendors" from less developed countries. So, for example, vendors in Turkey may be linked with recipients from Israel, or vendors from Brazil with recipients from the United States and surgeons in South Africa (Scheper-Hughes 2002b, 44–49). Reports of the prices paid by kidney recipients for their organs and the accompanying surgery and travel have varied, though the current "going rate" for a kidney is said to range from $10,000 to $20,000 (with the total cost to the recipients, including travel and hospital costs, at upwards of $200,000; see Friedlaender 2002, 972).[13] Most reports stress that very little of this money makes its way to the kidney vendors. Recent Iraqi donors, for example, probably received about $500 for a kidney (Friedlaender 2002, 971; see also Scheper-Hughes 2000).

While human rights groups and bioethicists have argued that these illegal markets simply point up the inequities that would result from legalized markets in organs, advocates of organ markets suggest that black markets are produced by the donation system, and would disappear in the presence of regulated organ compensation. Anderson and Barnett argue that illegal organ markets are the inevitable consequence of a donation system that cannot efficiently match supply and demand: "Economists unanimously agree that whenever authorities force lower-than-market prices upon a good or service, shortages and long lines develop. People at the back of the line often seek illegal or questionable alternatives" (Anderson and Barnett 1999, 1). In this view, markets will automatically form around "goods" such as organs (and services such as transplantation), and hindering the formation of a legal market will simply produce illegal markets. (Implicit in this claim is that illegal markets, while apparently more efficient than donation systems in matching supply and demand, are presumably not as efficient as legalized markets would be.) Thus while groups such as Organs Watch have noted that invariably organ "vendors" are desperately poor people, often inadequately advised on the health risks of their organ sales, economists such as Barnett, Beard, and Kaserman counter that the denial of compensation is "paternalistic in nature." They suggest that supporters of the current donation system simply substitute "moral or economic coercion" for organ donations in place of "the alleged 'economic coercion' that would accompany a market system" (Barnett, Beard, and Kaserman 1996, 670, 671).[14]

While opponents of organ markets often describe proposals for financial compensation as "neo-libertarian" in their goals, it is important to stress that in fact these proposals privilege precisely the same values of efficiency and equity that encouraged Congress to *forbid* organ sales in the early 1980s. Scheper-Hughes, for example, consistently characterizes organ market proposals as "a neo-liberal defense of individual rights" which privileges "individual rights" and "bodily autonomy" (Scheper-Hughes 2000, 197; see also Scheper-Hughes 2002a, 3). In similar fashion, Trevor Harrison sees market proposals as falling into two classes: libertarian arguments that stress people's right to "decide whether to alienate . . . their body," and "utilitarian arguments" that stress the outcome of organ markets, namely an increase in the supply of available organs (Harrison 1999, 31). While both Scheper-Hughes and Harrison are no doubt correct that neo-liberal and libertarian goals underpin many of the plans for organ sales, these proposals nevertheless appeal to values—efficiency and equity—that were associated with organ *donation* in hearings before Congress, and before that in Titmuss's more philosophical outline of blood "gifting."[15] These market advocates thus can justifiably position their critique as internal to the existing discourse on organ transplantation rather than an imposition of external values or criteria.

Organ Exchanges, eBay, and the Future of Community   The link between markets and real-time organ transplantation found symbolic expression in the late 1990s in the apparently unlikely venue of eBay, the well-known Internet auction site. On 26 August 1999 a purported vendor using the screen name "hchero" posted the following notice on the auction site: "Fully functional kidney for sale. You can choose either kidney. Buyer pays all transplant and medical costs. Of course only one for sale, as I need the other one to live. Serious bids only." Since eBay functions as an auction venue rather than an auctioneer per se (with rare exceptions, the vendor and not eBay decides what to sell, sets the range of acceptable prices, and warrants merchantability or authenticity), and because auction traffic on the site is so extensive (millions of transactions per day), by the time eBay officials became aware of the auction and pulled it (citing U.S. federal law, which forbids the sale of human organs), bids had reached $5.75 million.[16] Despite its unsuccessful conclusion, the story fascinated journalists, and accounts appeared in scores of newspapers and magazines worldwide. The event continues to be cited in the popular press as an extreme example of where the bold new world of e-commerce might lead (Cohen 2002, 210).

Both the ontological status of, and bids received for, hchero's kidney made it something of an anomaly on the eBay auction site. The explicit "use-value" of a kidney, for example, made it stand out from the usual items offered on eBay at the time, which generally had quite limited use-values: for example, old T-shirts, comic books, and knick-knacks. Most of these items have *some* use value—a comic book from the 1950s, for example, can still be read—but their exchange value (price) generally bore almost no relation to their utility; they were, from what we might call a strictly utilitarian view, useless. By contrast, a kidney seems to embody use-value itself: if, as Marx noted in *The German Ideology*, use-values and exchange values can only be produced when humans are "in a position to live," living itself requires the functioning body that supports this labor (Marx and Engels 1978, 155–56). The eBay kidney auction was also anomalous in that the amounts bid were far in excess of what a kidney was reputed to cost in the world's black markets. If John Frow found $200,000 for a kidney "somewhat improbable" in 1997, it is hard to know what superlative to use to describe a bid of $5.75 million (which was simply the last bid offered before the auction was terminated): $5.75 million would have bought more than two dozen kidneys even at the somewhat improbable price of $200,000. Bidding that overshot the "market price" by such an extreme margin was especially anomalous on eBay, which had notoriously depressed the price of collectibles for traditional dealers (since these dealers depended upon a lack of information flows about national and global prices, and eBay facilitated these flows).[17]

Commentators almost invariably have sought to explain these anomalies by describing the eBay kidney auction as a hoax (Harman 1999;

Cohen 2002, 210–11). Within the terms of this explanation, since there was no real kidney for auction, and because bidders must have recognized this, the item offered for sale could be anomalous, and the amounts wagered could be extreme, because in fact no real transaction was involved. "Hchero" was simply "playing" at being an organ seller, and eBay consumers were simply "playing" at being in the market for a kidney. While such sport might highlight the extent to which even commodification of human body parts seems funny (to some), it did not bear any relation to real organ markets (either the existing, illegal variety or possible future legal ones).[18]

While the eBay kidney auction may have been a hoax, to focus on this fact alone risks missing the ways in which this event brought into relief the intersection of organ markets and "speculative promise." There was, in other words, a striking "fit" between the eBay auction structure and proposals for organ markets. To begin with, the eBay site mirrored, in a rather uncanny way, the architecture of the organ transplantation information systems that had emerged in the 1980s and 1990s. As many congressional witnesses noted in the early 1980s, successful organ transplantation required the development of an extensive yet personalized computer system that could very rapidly match patients' histological profiles with available organs. While the development of such networks was still a difficult task in the mid-1980s, by the late 1990s the Internet had enabled them to develop almost on their own, and eBay was a prime example of this networking ability. The phenomenal financial success of eBay (it was one of the few Internet start-ups that turned a profit almost immediately) depended on creating a system that allowed the idiosyncrasies of consumer and seller to be matched. Although eBay dealt with purchasing, rather than histological, idiosyncrasies, it was clearly a network capable of the precise kinds of matching required by organ networks.

In addition, eBay's stress on "community values" seemingly provided a model for the ways in which organ markets could, *pace* their detractors, make "humanity more human." While eBay is a for-profit site that allows users to sell items to one another, it has always, and explicitly, positioned itself as a "community" that opposes the anonymity, greed, and suspicion of corporate and consumer culture, and the site emphasizes its purported commitment to these values both in its rhetoric and in its informational structure. A statement in the "Community Values" section of the web site reads: "eBay is a community where we encourage open and honest communication between all of our members." The site is said to be founded on "five basic values": "people are basically good"; "everyone has something to contribute"; "an honest, open environment can bring out the best in people"; everyone should be respected "as a unique individual"; and you should "treat others the way that you want to be treated."[19] Even the sales model—auctions rather than fixed prices—reinforces the notion of a community of committed enthusiasts rather than a faceless series of consumers. Thus, the eBay site not only mirrors the technical networking capacity of organ transplantation systems but purports to provide a quasi-market foundation for community values. In the terms posited by Callon (1998), eBay seeks to reentangle the disentangled world of commodity culture.

The attempted sale of an organ on the "community values" site eBay was a reminder of how "communities" and commodities are often also imbricated even in illegal organ sales. Most critics of organ sales charge that organ sales threaten to disentangle a formerly entangled system of organ donation, but both pro– and anti–organ market commentators (presumably for different reasons) have been unwilling to examine the extent to which the money for such sales itself emerges from, and facilitates, entangled communities. Scheper-Hughes provides one example of such entanglement in the case of the "Gruber" family from Israel, which worked with an organ broker ("Dr. F") to obtain a cadaveric kidney transplant from a clinic in the United States that was willing to ignore waiting lists in favor of patients with ready money. While some of the expense of the trip and organ transplantation was covered by the Grubers' insurance, "[t]he rest was raised through a private, but extensive, media campaign in Israel, which allowed this close-knit family of four to travel together to the USA for the duration of the eldest son's kidney transplant" (Scheper-Hughes 2002, 48). Such "private" gift communities are troubling in large part because they are not necessarily coterminous with national spaces, but follow other logics of association. EBay too follows a non-national logic of association, and its structurally decentralized and transnational commercial space provides a particularly compelling arena in which to work out the relationships between community, organs, and commerce.[20]

The most significant element of the "fit" between eBay and organ transplantation, however, is that an online auction site is the paradigm of an extremely efficient "real-time" market. The eBay information structure enables the flow of an enormous amount of information between buyers and sellers, and thus allows for the rapid and transparent establishment of market "equilibrium."[21] Yet by the same token, as the organ auction, whether real or hoax, demonstrated, it is equally capable of facilitating real-time market panics and "runs" on goods (and presumably services as well). In a sense, the kidney auction dramatizes the impossibility of regulating the fantasy of a regenerative body, bound up as it is with desire for mastery over time and the fear of death, through the rationalities of market forces. As Pixley (2004) notes, markets are the sites of powerful affects and desires, in which the ideal of rational equilibrium is readily subordinated to the distorting powers of fear, anxiety, and pleasure among both producers and consumers. This is all the more true of organ markets. Organs are not simple commodities but extremely complex forms of generative value that are not used and consumed in the usual sense but incorporated by the recipient as the condition of continuing life. Economists such as Blair and Kaserman have downplayed the possibility that organ markets could be plagued by cycles of glut and dearth, runs and bubbles, and various kinds of corporate corruption. Yet some of their own comparisons of organ markets to other industries do not inspire much faith in their claims. They suggest, for example, that organ markets might operate in ways analogous to markets for electric power (since both are "markets where either demand or supply is uncertain"; Blair and Kaserman 1991, 421–22), a comparison that should be greeted with some skepticism in the wake of the Enron scandal. Moreover, even with "futures" markets for cadaveric organs, there is every reason to expect the development of contract brokers, as well as the development of "derivatives" (i.e. rights to contracts) (Guttmann 1991, 460). As we have seen, a sense of entitlement to continuing life has become a feature of contemporary neoliberal, medical subjectivity. Hence the pricing signals sent by the market may have no purchase. For the wealthy on organ waiting lists, a kidney is literally priceless. In our analysis, the eBay auction plays out the difficulties of regulating such an unruly domain, where the excessive nature of demand constantly threatens to seek out illicit and exploitative sources of supply.

"Spare Parts," the Regenerative Body, and the Unlimited Demand for Organs The eBay organ auction, whether hoax or not, underscores that while pro-market organ economists have contributed significantly to our understanding of the various economic interests surrounding organ transplantation, their descriptions of the virtues of market efficiency depend upon the curiously unanalyzed claim that the "demand" for organs can in fact be fully satisfied. This claim stands at the moral center of many organ market proposals. To Barnett and Kaserman, for example, the only point of moving from a donation to a market system is to "eliminate the [organ] shortage" (Barnett and Kaserman 2000, 339), while Clay and Block claim that if organ transplantation "is turned over to the marketplace. . . . [e]veryone in need of an organ transplant will receive one" (Clay and Block 2002, 230).

Yet even a cursory glance at the statistics on transplant recipients in the United States suggests that the "demand" for organs is not constant, but ever-increasing.[22] The number of transplants performed in the United States rose from 12,619 in 1988 to 17,631 in 1993, 21,514 in 1998, and 25,468 in 2003.[23] As market advocates regularly insist, this increase in transplants performed is not the consequence of a well-functioning donation system, since in the same period the number of patients on waiting lists has grown much faster (as noted above, from 14,742 people in 1988 to 87,155 in 2004). This increase in both transplants and patients on waiting lists is in part a function of effective immunosuppressant drugs, which enable transplants for a greater number of patients. However, it is also due to an increase in what UNOS calls "repeat transplants" (that is, a second or third transplant for the same recipient), an increase in multiple-organ transplant procedures (such as heart and lung, or heart and lung and kidney), and an increase in the number of conditions for which transplantation is now considered viable.[24] In addition, more transplants are being performed on older patients. While in 1988 only 1.3 percent of all transplants in the United States went to patients over the age of 65 (and 2.9 percent to patients 50–64), by 2003, 11.9 percent of all transplants were for patients over the age of 65 (and 9.1 percent for patients 50–64).[25]

For a number of commentators, this increase in the number and kind of transplantations hints at a troubling moral shift in attitudes in the United States to life and medical progress. In the early 1990s, for example, Fox and Swazey argued that transplantation had become increasingly committed to "spare parts" pragmatism, the vision of the "replaceable body" and "limitless medical progress" (Fox and Swazey 1992, xv). Scheper-Hughes makes a similar point, arguing that this "scarcity [of organs], created by the technicians of transplant surgery, represents an artificial need, one that can never be satisfied, for underlying it is the unprecedented possibility of extending life indefinitely with the organs of others" (Scheper-Hughes 2000, 198). For Fox and Swazey the "spare parts" paradigm is a troubling sign of "our pervasive reluctance to accept the biological and human condition limits imposed by the aging process to which we are all subject and our ultimate mortality" (Fox and Swazey 1992, 204).

These analyses point to the centrality of certain fantasies about medical technology and its possibilities for perfecting the body and eliminating degeneration. These fantasies have evidently been nurtured inside transplant medicine. The field of regenerative medicine, discussed at various points throughout this book, has given a powerful impetus to these fantasies. As Brett Neilson notes, "With the discovery that the body does not age homogeneously, but unevenly replenishes cells and tissues in certain sites . . . the prospect of deploying genetic technologies to augment sites prone to degeneration (like the brain) and bringing them into line with self-renewing sites (like the bone marrow) feeds the dream of a completely regenerative biology" (Neilson 2003, 181). The dream of "a completely regenerative biology" has gained powerful institutional support in the United States from sources such as the Bayh-Dole legislation that we examined in chapter 3, and speculative personal tissue economies such as private cord-blood banking that we examined in chapter 4. In addition, the economic dependency of an aging population on speculative, regenerative technology has been powerfully underlined by the massive investment of pension funds in the biotech sector, tying future pension income to the success of these new medical technologies (Blackburn

2002; Neilson 2003; Cooper 2006). However, as many commentators have noted, regenerative medicine remains almost completely limited to in vitro technologies. It has yet to produce reliable or even experimental clinical applications (Neilson 2003; Hogle 2003; Cooper 2006). It seems to us that this speculation about the regenerative biology of the future puts a kind of "retrospective" pressure on "real-time" life-extending technologies, notably organ transplantation, which seeks regenerative capacities in the bodies of others. Frow succinctly describes this relationship between the fantasy of regeneration and the demand for organs: "Transplantation constructs a culturally very powerful myth of the social body—that is, of the limits and powers of all our bodies. This is the myth of the restoration of wholeness and of the integrity of the body: a myth of resurrection. Yet this wholeness can be achieved only by the incorporation of the other. The restored body is prostheticised: no longer an organic unity but constructed out of a supplement, an alien part which is the condition of that originary wholeness" (Frow 1997, 177). The fantasy of a regenerative body thus directs itself to the bodies of others, and creates a demand for new sites of tissue surplus. In the absence of a "national body" that can supply this demand—that is, in the absence of a sufficient number of fellow citizens willing to provide this surplus through the donation system—other possible sites of surplus become visible, for example third world bodies, national black markets, or legalized national (and international) markets. Harrison notes that the trade in organs "simply mirrors the 'normal' system of unequal exchanges that mark other forms of trade between the developed and undeveloped regions of the world" (Harrison 1999, 22). The poor in the South, unable to participate in the high-technology fantasy of endlessly renewable life, sell a portion of their body's capacities to wealthier patients in the North. "Spare" kidneys thus join the other flows of living, profitable matter (genetically or agriculturally valuable materials, human ova) that move from South to North to feed the demand for new forms of vitality and biovalue created by new biotechnologies (McNally and Wheale 1998).

Conclusion

THE FUTURE OF

TISSUE ECONOMIES

To draw together the strands of our analysis, we return to the questions that opened our account. What does it mean to give blood and other human tissues today, and what does it mean to receive them? What values and what kinds of embodied power relations are constituted by the exchange of human tissues, and what kind of social space does their circulation describe? The spectacular generosity of the blood donations after the World Trade Center attacks indicates that the idea of giving one's bodily tissues to restore the vitality of another is still highly compelling. It is evident from our investigations, however, that the social spaces constituted through the gift of tissues are quite different from the cohesive, inclusive, body politic of the welfare state posited by Titmuss. While Titmuss's imagined community of the tissue gift was highly idealized, it nevertheless based itself on the particularities of the western European postwar social contract, in which formal equality between citizens was underwritten by the state's provision of comprehensive social security. We have seen that the neoliberalization of this social contract has involved the deregulation and marketizing of some forms or aspects of human tissue economies, in the United Kingdom and to a greater degree in the United States, where the socialization of tissues was never comprehensive. The deregulation of tissue economies, and their proliferation and complication by new biotechnologies, has largely detached them from any image of a coherent national space and homogeneous population. The social spaces that they describe are more particular, more widely dispersed, and more susceptible to conflicts between different social actors over the degree and type of value inhering in tissues.

Certainly this deregulation has involved an increasing role for markets in the circulation of human tissues, a development that has led many commentators (Fox and Swazey 1992; Andrews and Nelkin 2001; Scheper-Hughes 2000; Scheper-Hughes 2002a; Gold 1996) to affirm the analytic and predictive power of Titmuss's gift-commodity dichotomy. In their analyses, once human tissues have exchange values and operate within some kind of market system they immediately lose the civil, humane powers of tissue exchange and instead reduce the human body to the level of thing and commodity. The only solution available in these analyses is the reaffirmation of the cohesive, regenerative power of the gift. However, our analysis of the field suggests that the form of the gift has no particular intrinsic powers of civil productivity, and offers no guarantees to protect the dignity of the donor or to produce benevolent sociality. The gift form has proved highly mutable and contextual as to its meaning, operation, and effects, and today it cannot function as a rejoinder or clear alternative to the incursion of market values into human tissue economies, for several reasons.

First, as tissue economies have become more complex, it is evident that the ideas of gift and commodity are inadequate to conceptualize exhaustively their *technicity*, and the ways this technicity mediates the values and relations associated with particular kinds of tissues. One crucial axis of technicity is that of entanglement and disentanglement —the ease or difficulty with which tissues can be accessed, multiplied, transformed, standardized, stored, and distributed; the extent to which they mimic currency and other forms of purely quantitative circulation. As we have seen, these qualities of entanglement and disentanglement stand in a complex and shifting relationship to the ontologizing of tissues, the degree to which they are taken to connote the person and dignity of the donor, and their aptness for gift or more commodified forms of circulation. Another axis of technicity is the extent to which the tissue circulates in a series of complex technical systems. We saw throughout the book that more disentangled tissues are more likely to move through transformations, global sites, and various regulatory regimes, and hence are open to nonpredictable interactions, risk events, and singularities. This axis in particular demonstrates that tissue gifts have no essential powers to confer vitality. Gifts circulating through such systems can be readily transformed into bad gifts, contaminants. The blood contamination scandals of the 1980s, the current anxieties about vCJD in the blood supply in Britain, and the general public perception in Europe and the United States that the blood supply is intrinsically a source of disease have developed because blood flows through such complex technical systems, and interacts with so many bodies in ways that become incalculable. Rather than a form of circulation that includes all citizens and revivifies the body politic, it has become a form of circulation that divides populations precisely because it links them: that is, the capacity for biological linkages between "infected" body fragments and "healthy" individuals enables populations to imagine themselves as clean and other populations as contaminated. The power of the gift to circulate tissues potentially vitiates rather than augments the body politic. Donor pools shrink, patients elect to have autologous blood transfusion, and the gift of blood becomes something to avoid, except when personal or collective emergencies (car accident, terrorist attack) override lesser considerations of risk.

Second, the status of the tissue gift has fundamentally altered with the rapid expansion of the for-profit biotechnology sector. The current cycle of expansion in finance capital (Arrighi 1994) has exploited bodily processes in unprecedented ways, constituting the biological productivity of in vitro tissues as a site for profitable investment (Cooper 2006). As Blackburn (2002) has noted, a significant amount of the venture capital that has propelled for-profit biotechnology stems either directly or indirectly from national pension funds, especially those of the United Kingdom and the United States. This complicates considerably the relationship between national tissue economies and the globalization of tissue flows, as the pension funds designed to safeguard the welfare of an aging national body politic have effectively become the means for further disentangling particular tissues and samples from their national origins.

The tissues employed as "speculative" assets by corporations such as Sandoz Pharmaceutical and Geron originate in the bodies of patients or citizen-donors, who effectively act as an open source of free "raw material" through various systems of gratuitous gifting. Once removed from the body, human tissues are less and less likely to remain within a gift system, and more likely to end up in commercial research and development laboratories, undergoing profitable transformations. This change is not simply the alternation of a gift with a commodity status, the emergence of a simple mixed economy, but rather involves the historical modification of both forms of value. As we saw in chapters 2 and 3, from the point of view of intellectual property law, the donor's gift is another form of waste tissue, analogous to the tissue abandoned in the clinic, without value before its appropriation and technical and legal improvement. The expansion of informed consent procedures for tissue donation in the United Kingdom does not function as a means for endowing abandoned tissue with the recuperative powers of the gift, but rather serves to transform waste tissues into commodities. As we argued in chapter 2, informed consent procedures have become a way to free donated tissues from the donor's claims, and make them available for appropriation and the establishment of commercial intellectual property rights. At the same time, as Cooper (2006) and Strathern (1999) note, intellectual property is not a simple commodity form, an immediate exchange value on a market, but rather a speculative value, a form of property-in-ideas whose value takes place in the future. So in this modified tissue economy, gift and waste tissues are equivalent rather than opposite values, and both are transformed through biotechnical intervention into *a material idea* whose value is generated by being deferred. The advent of speculative value into tissue economies thus introduces a fourth term, which further disables the apparent clarity of the gift-commodity distinction.

However, we also saw that the property relations generated through intellectual property are highly variable, and do not necessarily involve the exclusivity of access and disposal implied in the classic notion of private property. While donors themselves are certainly excluded from personal intellectual property rights in their tissues, intellectual property rights within the research domain can be configured in different ways. Many biotechnical researchers in both the public and private sectors are committed to maintaining an open-source biocommons, a public domain, exemplified by the Human Genome Project, where basic research and research tools are retained as public property, and where patent licenses are differentially priced or waived to favor certain kinds of public-good research. Here intellectual property can be configured to create permeabilities between public and private knowledge, and ensure a degree of gratuitous circulation between researchers and clinicians. We also saw the development of particular patient-researcher relations built up around intellectual property. Patient organizations and private medical charities like the Juvenile Diabetes Research Foundation and the Christopher Reeve Foundation are increasingly involved in both funding and guiding for-profit research (Rabinow 1999; Hogle 2004). The evolution of these alliances between civil society and commercial interests may well see further adaptations of patent as a way to express research partnerships.

Furthermore, the establishment of intellectual property in tissues does not necessarily require marketizing them at the point of distribution as transplantable tissue or pharmaceutical regime. A number of forces can intervene to retain patented tissues and their research yields at a point of common access. We saw that the UK Stem Cell Bank is establishing itself as an obligatory passage point through which all stem cell materials and research in the United Kingdom must pass, where public sector researchers can gain access to materials for marginal costs, and where any resultant therapies will be retained within the public domain of the National Health Service. In short, while at the point of donation donors are increasingly dispossessed, the appropriation of their tissues as intellectual property does not dictate for-profit delivery downstream. State intervention can resocialize research results and therapeutic applications, which our research suggests will be important in maintaining the flow of embryonic gifts in the stem cell area in the United Kingdom. Here we can see a decisive difference between tissue economies in the United States and the United Kingdom that seems likely to obtain in the future—the commitment to a national health system in the United Kingdom gives the state strong incentives to fund interim institutions like the Stem Cell Bank, and to manage tissue economies in such a way that the costs of therapeutic delivery do not go beyond the means of the National Health Service.

Finally, we consider that the form of the gift is mutating in response to a fundamental shift in social relations and in the medical technologies used for regenerating the bodies of populations. *The Gift Relationship* can be read as a proposal for constituting both the health of the population and the social cohesion of the welfare state through the redistribution of generative biological matter—from those bodies who can afford to give (because they are healthy and can regenerate their blood) to those in need. Cooper (2006) argues that the biotechnology revolution of the 1980s signaled a major shift in the sociotechnical basis for health production and biological regeneration. It involved a major incursion of capital markets into the task of biological regeneration, focusing not on redistributive relations between citizens but on the diversion of human tissues through laboratory processes aimed at investing it with a speculative surplus of life" (Cooper 2006). The field of regenerative medicine, encompassing the most recent tissue economies—stem cell technologies, tissue engineering, the use of growth factors—is precisely concerned with experimenting with the body's own capacity for surplus growth (Cooper 2006).

While regenerative medicine potentiates allogenic tissue networks (like embryonic stem cell networks), we have identified the emergence of autologous tissue economies based on the promise of regenerative medicine as a further innovation in tissue values. Autologous services have grown up around peripheral blood, cord blood, and reproductive tissue (ovarian tissue can be banked for use after cancer therapy, for example), and we anticipate that with further developments in the technologies of regenerative medicine, such autologous services will expand. We have analyzed this growth in autologous services as one response to the politicizing of allogenic tissue networks, because of contamination and retention scandals, donor shortages, and regulatory difficulties in the face of globalized tissue economies. They serve to withdraw the donor from the risks of allogenic tissue economies, and promise to locate surpluses of vitality within the patient's own body, rather than in a social surplus. Regenerative medicine promises that the body can become the source of its own self-renewal, an attractive prospect for aging populations. This autologous economy does not depend on either a gift or a commodity form in the strict sense, but rather involves the strategic investment of a part of the donor's body in a biotechnical venture, whose payoff will be biological self-enhancement rather than financial reward or civil renewal.

At the same time, the interregnum between the ever-deferred promise of regenerative medicine and the contemporary fantasy of a regenerative body, open to endless renewal, has produced a voracious demand for more established forms of organ transplant. As waiting lists for organs lengthen, the wealthy seek tissues elsewhere, in the bodies of the poor in developing nations. As the blood contamination scandals remind us, the poor, lacking the hope of an extended life span, can be readily inveigled into spending their bodies in the present.[1] Hence the South readily appears as a source of tissue surplus for the North. The dizzy bids during the eBay kidney auction suggest (perhaps satirically?) the intensity of consumer desire that drives the global black markets for human organs and tissues and the kinds of cash available to disentangle the most recalcitrant of human tissues—solid, non-renewable organs—from the bodies of the poor. Here we can see that the wealthy can purchase the fantasy of a regenerative body at the expense of the health of other, less valuable bodies.

As we stated at the outset, tissue economies are at base about the way the biological capacities of the human body contribute to social, economic, and political systems of productivity and power. At the macroeconomic level, the present biopolitical situation appears to be riven with inequity and nonreciprocal forms of economy. The surplus profit and biovalue generated by commercial biotechnology innovation depend on the dispossession of donors, while the wealthy in the North secure their health and longevity at the expense of the bodies of the poor in the South. At the same time, our map of contemporary tissue economies has identified mitigating forces in new sites of consultation and regulation (for example the Stem Cell Bank and the foreshadowed Human Tissue Authority) and local forms of negotiation and innovation (for example the emerging alliances between patient groups and medical researchers). The tenor of these mitigating forces in a sense mirrors the national differences highlighted by Titmuss.

The United Kingdom has turned to nationally oriented, regulatory solutions to the problems of disentanglement (such as the Stem Cell Bank), while many of the more compelling solutions that have emerged in the United States attempt to work within existing commercial and property structures (such as the use of gene patents by PXE International).[2] However, in both cases it is clear that the old gift-commodity distinction is quite unable to encompass the complexities of these hybrid and often microeconomic arrangements. It seems to us that these are the sites where future contestations and negotiations over the biopolitical economy of human tissues will take place.

Notes

Introduction

1 A series of studies of the volume of blood collection in the United States (Wallace et al. 1995; Wallace et al. 1998; Sullivan et al. 2002) reveals a steady decline throughout the late 1980s and 1990s, and an ever-narrowing margin of collections over transfusions.

2 Blood transfusion has been sporadically practiced since the seventeenth century in Europe, but it has only been a routine procedure since the early twentieth century, when the classification of blood types and the development of anticoagulant made transfusion safer and more effective. The early procedure was to transfuse blood directly between donor and patient as they lay side by side in the clinic. There were no techniques for storing blood until the Spanish Civil War.

3 In 1951, for example, the Red Cross was "designated as the Government's blood collection agency for defense purposes—both military and civil defense" (Dr. Sam Gibson, in U.S. Congress 1964, 62). It should be noted that civilian disasters, such as plane crashes, will also elicit a surge in blood donors (Schmidt 2002), although such events do not produce the same donor-to-recipient ratio as was evident in the attacks on the World Trade Center.

4 See Kaldor 1999 for the transformation of war from a struggle between the standing armies of nation-states to internecine conflicts between globalized religious and ethnic diasporas.

5 The American Red Cross found itself embroiled in a scandal after the terrorist attack because it did not pay sufficient attention to the particularity of donations. The massive outpouring of blood donations was equaled by cash donations to the Red Cross's "Liberty Fund," a fund established in the days after the disaster which eventually received $967

million. Within a month the "Liberty Fund" had come under fire after the Red Cross disclosed that the donated funds were in fact not specifically set aside for the World Trade Center attacks and that much of the money was slotted for corporate needs such as improvements to the Red Cross's telecommunication systems. Red Cross officials claimed that it had never been their policy to allow contributors to earmark their donations for a specific disaster, but the scandal became so intense that the federal government conducted hearings into the propriety of the Red Cross's actions. Its chief executive officer, Dr. Bernadine Healy, attempted to redefine the Liberty Fund as a more long-term "war fund," aligning it with President George Bush's declared war on terrorism, but many donors remained angry and unconvinced: just as blood donors were insistent on donating blood *now*, for *this* emergency (rather than waiting for several months when supplies would again presumably decline), so too were monetary donors unwilling to see their gifts attenuated by being converted into a long-term war fund. In the wake of this criticism, the Red Cross altered its policy, allowing the Liberty Fund to be directed specifically to the disaster. For a few of numerous newspaper accounts see www.cnn.com/2001/US/11/06/rec.charity.hearing/?related and www.cbsnews.com/stories/2002/06/05/national/main511125.shtml; accessed 1 June 2003.

6 See for example www.nature.com/nsu/030421/030421-2.html.

7 See for example Barnett, Beard, and Kaserman (1993), who examine the deleterious effects that the nonremunerated status of organs has on hospital budgeting procedures; and Peters (1991), who argues for a death benefit to be paid to the family as a way to increase organ procurement. For analytic discussions of the logic of this position see Munzer 1994 and Joralemon 2000.

8 The IEA's ideas strongly influenced Thatcher's radical deregulation of the economy in the 1980s. For a full account of the debates between Titmuss and the IEA see Fontaine 2002.

9 Sperm "donation" is one persistent exception to this rule. Sperm donors in most countries are paid a fee, although it is sometimes described as reimbursement for expenses.

10 See www.scandinaviancryobank.com.

Chapter 1: Blood Banks, Risk, and Autologous Donation

1 See for example Nuffield Council on Bioethics, *Human Tissue: Ethical and Legal Issues* (April 1995); Working Party of the Royal College of Pathologists and the Institute of Biomedical Science, *Consensus Statement of*

Recommended Policies for Uses of Human Tissue in Research, Education and Quality Control (1999); and Medical Research Council, *Working Group on Human Tissue and Biological Samples for Use in Research: Report of the Medical Research Council Working Group to Develop Operational and Ethical Guidelines* (1999).

2 The situation in Britain was slightly more complicated. The NBS was set up as part of the National Health Service but its remit was limited to England and Wales, as Scotland set up an autonomous service.

3 Hemophilia is a genetic condition whose sufferers, always male, lack a blood-clotting protein. Untreated, hemophilia involves the continued risk of fatal bleeding incidents, frequent, painful bleeds into the joints, and an early death.

4 Rabinow (1999) describes the rejection of an article to that effect by the *New England Journal of Medicine* in 1982 on the grounds of insufficient proof and the potential to cause alarm.

5 In France blood industry executives were imprisoned in the wake of widespread HIV infection of the blood supply, and three government officials, including the former prime minister Laurent Fabius, were tried for manslaughter. Only one, the former health minister Edmond Hervé, was convicted.

6 The term "serum hepatitis" was used in the 1960s and 1970s to describe what are now recognized as hepatitis B and C, forms of blood-borne hepatitis transmitted through the blood supply. At the time Titmuss was writing, a test for hepatitis B existed, but hepatitis C was not identified until 1989.

7 In Australia the situation was reversed. In early 1983 the Sydney Blood Transfusion Service unilaterally banned gay male donors from giving blood, and by 1984 donors were required to declare in writing that they had not engaged in male-to-male sexual activity over the last five years.

8 Blood donors cannot contract infection, because of nonreusable donation packs that include their own syringe.

9 See www.info.doh.gov.uk/doh/embroadcast.nsf/vwDiscussionAll/ 0301ECC6DF485EF880256 DFF004DA063.

Chapter 2: Disentangling the Embryonic Gift

1 For an extended critique of this idea see Waldby and Squier 2003.

2 Immortalized human cell lines have been important technologies in medical research since the 1950s, and today thousands of human tissue cell lines are in use throughout the world (Lock 2001).

3 The Human Genetics Advisory Commission Report on cloning (1998) found that a number of those whom it consulted found the distinction between therapeutic and reproductive cloning arbitrary and meaningless.

4 See Medical Research Council Press Releases, "First Stem Cell Lines to Be Deposited as UK Stem Cell Bank Officially Opens Today" (19 May 2004) and "MRC Appoints National Institute for Biological Standards and Control to Set Up UK Stem Cell Bank" (9 September 2002), available at www.mrc.ac.uk; accessed 12 August 2004.

5 Personal communication with the director of the UK Stem Cell Bank.

6 Catherine Waldby would like to thank Celia Lury for bringing this article to her attention.

7 In these terms, it is not surprising that before the anonymizing of organ donation, donor families and recipients would find themselves in what Fox and Swazey (1992) describe as quasi-kinship relations, in which donor families take a proprietary interest in the behavior of the recipient, and recipients feel too grateful and guilty to protest.

8 Including Nuffield Council on Bioethics, *Human Tissue: Ethical and Legal Issues* (April 1995); Working Party of the Royal College of Pathologists and the Institute of Biomedical Science, *Consensus Statement of Recommended Policies for Uses of Human Tissue in Research, Education and Quality Control* (1999); and Medical Research Council, *Working Group on Human Tissue and Biological Samples for Use in Research: Report of the Medical Research Council Working Group to Develop Operational and Ethical Guidelines* (1999).

9 Part II of this book—Waste and Tissue Economies—deals with the "abandoned" tissue, which is not actively given but passively surrendered as part of a surgical or other procedure.

10 In that case, in which Kelly, an artist, had taken body parts from the anatomy rooms of the Royal College of Surgeons, the court found "an exception to the traditional common law rule that 'there is no property in a corpse,' namely, that once a human body or body part has undergone a process of skill by a person authorized to perform it, with the object of preserving for the purpose of medical or scientific examination or for the benefit of medical science, it becomes something quite different from an interred corpse. It thereby acquires a usefulness or value. It is capable of becoming property in the usual way, and can be stolen." Regina v. Kelly, 1999 QB 621 (C.A.).

11 Steering Committee of the UK Stem Cell Bank (2004), annex 2a, "Donor Information and Consent Form."

12 Totipotent cells give rise to both the embryo itself and the placenta and supporting tissue.

13 UK Patent Office Notices, April 2003, available at www.patent.gov. uk/patent/notices/practice/stemcells.htm; accessed 13 January 2005.

14 See also Lock 2001 on this case.

15 The study, of public perceptions of stem cell technologies and the stem cell bank, involved focus group research with twelve groups in eight English towns, including six groups of men and women with direct experience of IVF.

16 Steering Committee of the UK Stem Cell Bank (2004), annex 2a, "Donor Information and Consent Form."

17 Set out in Steering Committee of the UK Stem Cell Bank (2004), annex 11, "Terms and Conditions for Deposition and Access of Human Stem Cell Lines."

Part II: Waste and Tissue Economies

1 See http://www.atcc.org.

Chapter 3: The Laws of Mo(o)re

1 Whether this is true is still an open question. In *Body Bazaar* Andrews and Nelkin point to several studies suggesting that proprietary claims in tissue types, research procedures, and genetic information in fact have cut down considerably on the flow of information between institutions and laboratories. See Andrews and Nelkin 2001, 5, 55.

2 There was, moreover, a certain irony in the Court's faith in the UCLA infectious waste disposal system, since congressional hearings in 1988 had highlighted potential problems with infectious waste disposal systems in the United States, for example the possibility that incineration was producing cancer-causing dioxins and furans. The hearings were initiated in the wake of heavily publicized accounts of medical waste washing up on the shores of New York and New Jersey, though it subsequently was determined that little of this waste came from hospitals (Manns 1995, 547; Harrell and Catanzariti 1994, 2).

3 The California Supreme Court dismissed the very different reading of "abandonment" provided by the Court of Appeal. In its decision the Court of Appeal had held that Moore's consent to have his spleen removed had not constituted "abandonment": "[t]he essential element of abandonment is the intent to abandon," for "[t]he owner of the property abandoned must be 'entirely indifferent as to what may become of it or as to who may thereafter possess it' " (*Moore v. U. of Cal.* 1988, 41, 509). The court thus concluded that a "consent to removal of a diseased organ, or the taking of blood or other bodily tissues, does not necessarily imply an intent to abandon such organ, blood or tissue" (*Moore v. U. of Cal.* 1988, 41, 509).

4 Such ontological ambiguity points to the difficulty of trying to address this case through either existing critical commodity or waste theories. While Arjun Appadurai's notion of the "commodity situation" captures the ways in which the status of an object can shift between categories such as "gift," "barter-object," and "object of monetary exchange," depending on context, it is not clear that the notion helps us to understand how the categories of gift and commodity are aligned with the ontological transformations (from diseased spleen to immortal cell line) at play in this case (Appadurai 1986). In similar fashion, Michael Thompson's "rubbish theory" provides a compelling explanation of the cycles by means of which objects move between the categories "transient" (in which their value decreases) to "rubbish" (in which they hold no value) to "durable" (in which their value increases), but his theory too assumes a stable object (for example, consumer items such as a car or real estate) (Thompson 1979).

5 In its majority opinion the California Supreme Court also suggested that creating a cell line was an "art," citing a publication by the Office of Technology Assessment (OTA) entitled *New Developments in Biotechnology* as support for this claim, as well as most of its other claims about technical aspects of cells and cell line creation (*Moore v. U. of Cal.* 1990, 127 n. 2). The court's decision to cite this OTA report was in some sense peculiar, for the report itself—published after the initial decision in *Moore* by the California Superior Court but before the Court of Appeal had rendered its verdict— had used the *Moore* case as one of four examples of the ethical difficulties attending biocommerce (U.S. Congress, Office of Technology Assessment 1987, 26ff). The California Supreme Court thus derived its factual knowledge about cell lines from a document that suggested that the very case under review was one of the keys to the future of biotechnology.

6 We take the term "climate" from the Bayh-Dole hearings, considered later in this chapter. For an example of this term see U.S. Congress 1980b, 19.

7 In *Shamans, Software, and Spleens*, James Boyle argues that these two rationales seem to work at cross-purposes, since the court finds itself claiming on the one hand that property rights in cells will impede the flow of information, and on the other hand that the production of information requires that someone be granted property right in cells (Boyle 1996, 24). We are not so sure that this is a contradiction, though, because the court seems to be implying a complicated ecology between three different types of bodies. There is, first, the individual "dignified" human body and, second, a dignified "body of information" that is produced by research institutions. Both of these must be kept pure, but they can maintain their dignity only if *corporate* bodies (who have already submitted to the profane economic world) labor in the sewers of commerce. The body of information mediates between these other two bodies (individual and corporate), with "waste" serving as the rhetorical technology that keeps individual bodies dignified.

8 It is not entirely clear whether the "innocent parties" to be protected were researchers who employed human cell lines, or patients who indirectly benefited from that research. However, this ambiguity fits perfectly the logic of the majority decision, which suggests at every point that these two interests are always aligned.

9 U.S. Congress 1984a, 110. See also 1, 11, 76, and 117. In the third and final hearing, Chairman Waxman was more specific, contending that "three out of four Americans would donate if given the chance" (287).

10 See U.S. Congress 1976; U.S. Congress 1978a; U.S. Congress 1978b; U.S. Congress 1980a; U.S. Congress 1980b.

11 This number had expanded to thirty thousand by 1980, apparently additional proof of government waste (U.S. Congress 1980a, 538). Yet few members of Congress were interested in how that level of government patent "waste" corresponded to levels of patent "waste" in private corporations (for a rare attempt to pursue this line of questioning see U.S. Congress 1976, 80). For recent critiques of the applicability of these statistics to the question of government patenting efficiency, see Eisenberg 1996 and Mowery et al. 2004, 91.

12 This was the description by Senator Russell B. Long of Louisiana of the Schmitt-Stevenson Bill, which was almost identical to the Bayh-Dole Act.

13 So, for example, of all DNA patents issued between 1980 and 1993, 39 percent went to "academic institutions," a label that includes public universities, private universities, nonprofit institutes and hospitals, and government institutions (McCormack and Cook-Deegan 1999). However, it is also important to recognize that university patenting in the United States had already increased sharply in the early 1970s, especially in the arena of biomedicine, and several major universities had begun to campaign for patent reform before the introduction of Bayh-Dole (Mowery et al. 2004, 46–47, 55–56). Thus as Mowery et al. (2004) note, "Bayh-Dole is properly viewed as initiating the latest, rather than the first, phase in the history of U.S. university patenting."

14 We suggest that philosophically oriented commentators such as Hans Jonas and Curtis R. Naser have missed the mark when they argue that the "good of society" should not be conflated with medical progress. Naser, for example, argues that "[b]iomedical research . . . is not a good that in itself is necessary to the continuation of the state or the maintenance of the orderly fabric of society" (Naser 1998, 170), and Jonas argues that "medical progress is an optional goal, not an unconditional commitment" (cited in Naser 1998, 170). While this may be true in an abstract sense, it entirely misses the extent to which Bayh-Dole legislation tied national existence (or at least competitive advantage) to "progress" in the form of innovation in fields such as biomedicine.

15 The *Moore* case was cited, for example, in a California trial as part of a strategy to block a woman's attempt to take possession of her dead boyfriend's frozen sperm (Boulier 1995, 693–731). As Sealing notes, it is important to recognize that courts have failed to follow the Moore precedent in different senses, some "declin[ing] to adopt its fiduciary duty standard," others ruling that physicians should not have to disclose commercial interests even to the limited extent mandated by the California Supreme Court (Sealing 2002, 758–59). We also note that five states (Alaska, Colorado, Florida, Georgia and Louisiana)—perhaps in response to the *Moore* decision—"explicitly define genetic information as personal property" (see the National Conference of State Legislatures web site, http://www.ncsl.org/programs/health/genetics/prt.htm; accessed 4 December 2004). The legal implications of these very recent state laws are not at all clear and have yet to be tested. (Thanks to Lauren Dame for this information.)

Chapter 4: Umbilical Cord Blood

1 See the web site of the National Marrow Donor Program (USA), http://www.marrow.org; accessed 29 March 2004.

2 Ibid.

3 See Cancer Research UK website, www.cancerresearchuk.org/; accessed 9 October 2003.

4 See the web site of the National Marrow Donor Program (USA), http://www.marrow.org; accessed 13 January 2004.

5 At the time of writing cord-blood banking in the United Kingdom was regulated by the Department of Health Code of Practice for Tissue Banking and the Human Tissue Act of 2004. The department's code of practice will be superseded in 2006 by European Directive 2004/23/EC on "setting standards of quality and safety for the donation, procurement, testing, processing, preservation, storage and distribution of human tissues and cells."

6 The Food and Drug Administration regulates public cord-blood banking in the United States, but its jurisdiction over private banks is unclear and contested. See Fredrickson 1998 for an account of some of this contestation. Private cord-blood banks must now register and list with the FDA, and some states have mandatory licensing and regulation for quality assurance.

7 See web site of the National Marrow Donor Program (USA), http://www.marrow.org; accessed 29 March 2004.

8 At the time of writing, four private banks operated in the United Kingdom: the UK Cord Blood Bank, Cryo-Care, Future Health Europe, and Cells4Life.

9 See www.mtsinai.on.ca/cord_blood/faq; accessed 31 December 2003.

10 For a further sample of excerpts from various medical peak organizations' opinions on this matter see Comité Consultatif National d'Ethique 2002.

11 See www.mtsinai.on.ca/cord_blood/faq; accessed 31 December 2003.

12 See www.lifebank.com/parents/questions; accessed 12 March 2003.

13 Interview with Ron Penny for the program "Catalyst," Australian Broadcasting Service Television, 25 September 2003.

14 See www.mtsinai.on.ca/cord; accessed 13 February 2003.

15 Interview for the program "Catalyst" with the father of a child whose cord blood had been banked at Cryocite, Australian Broadcasting Service Television, 25 September 2003.

16 "Potent Stem Cells Found in Baby Teeth," http://ScientificAmerican.com, 23 April 2003; accessed 12 September 2004.

Chapter 5: Commodity-Communities

1 Both quotes taken from http://www.law.duke.edu/news/current/20020905pdic.html; accessed 9 January 2003.

2 See http://usinfo.state.gov/topical/global/biotech/00031401.htm; accessed 9 January 2003.

3 In *Common Field and Enclosure in England, 1450–1850* (1977, unnumbered Preface page), A. Yelling also notes that the period 1907–15 was characterized by intense interest in the history of the commons and enclosure.

4 The authors of *Whose Common Future?* suggest that the loss of traditional commons was the necessary precondition for the rise of "empires and states, business conglomerates and civic dictatorships" (Ecologist 1993, 21). See also Rose 1986, 742, and for a useful summary of critical approaches to the definition and practices of commons, see Butler 1982 and the list in Lessig 2001, 271 n. 1.

5 See General Assembly resolution 2749 (XXV) of 17 December 1970. This movement had an interesting Lockean precedent: Locke noted that "amongst those who are counted the civilized part of mankind, who have made and multiplied positive laws to determine property, this original law of Nature for the beginning of property, in what was before common, still takes place, and by virtue thereof, what fish any one catches in the ocean, that great and still remaining common of mankind" (Locke 1988, I:29). For a useful survey of concepts of the global commons see Joyner 2001, Ostrom 1990, and Baslar 1998.

6 It is also worth noting that this first version of the biomedical commons was characterized by the "regionalism" described as typical of the commons. Fox and Swazey highlight how the "norms" governing local biomedical commons were exclusionary, noting that the Northwest Kidney Center in Seattle, for example, created a committee "composed of responsible middle class and upper-middle class members of the community" to decide which patients on transplant lists should receive organs, yet the committee's "selection criteria were, at times, shaped by their largely subliminal views of 'social worth'" (Fox and Swazey 1992, 82).

7 The proposed Collections of Information Anti-Piracy Act even positions public domain works such as Shakespeare's plays as "data" in this sense.

8 So, for example, the Copyright Term Extension Act of 1998 has, at least in the eyes of some legal scholars, created "perpetual copyright" (Samuelson 2001, 87–88 n. 27).

9 This is Samuelson's definition of the "public domain," which she equates with the commons.

10 See for example the web sites of the Open Bioinformatics Foundation (http://www.open-bio.org), BIOS (www.bios.com), Creative Commons (http://creativecommons.org), the Electronic Frontier Foundation (www.eff.org), Public Knowledge (http://www.publicknowledge.org/about-us/mission-statement.html), and UW BioCommons (http://bio commons.bcc.washington.edu).

11 We also note that the "information commons" has a more expansive range of contents than the public domain. The latter has traditionally been tied to notions of "high culture" (for example the works of Shakespeare), while theories of the information commons have tended to highlight both shared cultural and technical artifacts (for example the works of Shakespeare and gene sequence data). The relationship between the information commons and the public sphere is more complicated. Frow has noted that "all uses of the commons implicate in one way or another the concept of the public sphere" (Frow 1997, 212).

12 See Crichton (1990) and the film *Jurassic Park* (Stephen Spielberg, Universal, 1995). In Michael Crichton's novel the park's bioengineered dinosaurs were all created female to ensure de facto sterility. To the surprise of the bioengineers, however, the dinosaurs quickly acquire the ability to breed uncontrollably. This is represented as a direct consequence of bioengineering methodology: the engineers, able to extract only fragmentary bits of dinosaur DNA from mosquitoes preserved in amber, decided to "complete" these DNA fragments with frog DNA; however, the frog DNA imparted to the dinosaurs the ability to change sex in "environment[s] in which all the animals are of the same sex" (Crichton 1990, 373). The voice of prudence in the novel (Ian Malcolm) contends that this is simply an example of a more general capacity of "life" "[t]o be unpredictable" (284).

13 While we are not aware that Shiva herself uses the image of the dinosaur in her discussions of biodiversity and biopiracy, the image nevertheless appears frequently in discussions of indigenous rights and the project of reclaiming the commons. As W. J. T. Mitchell notes in *The Last Dinosaur Book: The Life and Times of a Cultural Icon*, dinosaurs are images central to discussions of capitalism, serving as a symbol of "the cycle of innovation and obsolescence that is central to the logic of both modern science and technology and modern capitalism" (Mitchell 1998, 88) but also of "the fate of the human species within the world system of modern capitalism" (67). An example of the intersection of these two symbols is found in James Meek's and Paul Brown's "Patenting Life: How US Muscle Bent the Rules in Europe" in the *Guardian*, in which they contend that the patent system in Europe is in disarray because the European Patent Office "is a dinosaur, left over from an earlier age of European cooperation" (Meek and Brown 2000). The result of leaving a "dinosaur" in charge of patents, they contend, is an expansion of European patent protection over life forms, a step that has serious—and perhaps even globally fatal—consequences.

14 As Hayden (2003) has noted, "bioprospecting" is a complicated term, also employed by academic researchers who profess to *support* the claims and rights of indigenous peoples by providing them with benefit-sharing agreements. Hayden contends that such attempts to position indigenous groups as "stakeholders" have the effect, intended or not, of (re)locating indigenous knowledge within a neoliberal framework.

15 For a brief, and critical, discussion of the assumptions that underpin many of the open-source bioinformatics processing tools, see Thacker 2004, 57–59.

16 A small number of critics deny that strictly monetary incentives are necessary for innovation, and point to other factors, such as prestige and awards, that could take the place of intellectual property rights. As proof that these methods would work, they point to the continuing production of free music files, open-source computer programs such as Linux, the open-source genomics project (www.ensembl.org), and so on. More sophisticated analyses illuminate how monetary and nonmonetary incentives work in conjunction with one another (Lerner and Tirole 2002; Mustonen 2003). Thus, for example, contributors to open-source communities generate prestige that can be translated into consultancies (Mustonen 2003).

17 Quote from "The General Public License (G PL)" section of the Open Source web site, http://www.opensource.org/licenses/gpl-license.php.

18 Affymetrix has made its position clear in public talks, such as that given in 2002 at Duke University at the symposium "Commercialization of Human Genomics: Consequences for Science and Humanity," and more implicitly through its web site, which in a section entitled "For the educator" provides links to a number of position papers on "patenting DNA," almost all of which argue against it. The documents linked to this part of the site are documents from the Duke symposium itself; a discussion paper of the Nuffield Council on Bioethics entitled "The Ethics of Patenting DNA"; "The Genetic Age: Who Owns the Genome," a webcast event sponsored by Affymetrix, as well as a review paper of the event by the John Marshall Law School; patent guidelines provided by the Biotechnology Industry Organization (BIO); and "Who Owns the Genome? Human Genetics and Intellectual Property," a discussion hosted by the Forum on Technology and Innovation.

19 Quote from the symposium "Commercialization of Human Genomics: Consequences for Science and Humanity" presented at the Duke University Center for Genome Ethics, Law, and Policy, 27 September 2002, webcast available at http://www.law.duke.edu/conference/gelp/program.html.

20 For more information about this corporation and its activities see its web site at http://www.PXE.org. Our claims are based primarily on personal communications with the Terrys, but all of these points are substantiated in the Terrys' presentations about PXE International in the fall of 2002 at the symposium "Commercialization of Human Genomics: Consequences for Science and Humanity," archived at the web site of the Duke University Center for Genome Ethics, Law, and Policy, http://www.law.duke.edu/conference/gelp/program.html.

21 Quote taken from a Power Point slide in Sharon Terry's presentation at the symposium "Commercialization of Human Genomics: Consequences for Science and Humanity," Duke University Center for Genome Ethics, Law, and Policy, fall 2002, webcast available at http://www.law.duke.edu/ conference/gelp/program.html.

22 Shiva suggests, for example, that "[n]on-Western medical systems. . . . might not exchange their knowledge freely, [but] they do freely gift its benefits" (Shiva 1997, 68).

Chapter 6: Real-Time Demand

1 For an account of the two physicians who attempted to serve as organ brokers, see the *Guardian*, 20 October 2002.

2 Contrary to our treatment of the subject, some commentators argue that tissues and organs connote legally, medically, and arguably even ontologically separate categories, and have suggested that these distinctions lead to fundamentally different economies. According to the anthropologist Lesley Sharp, for example, "[o]ne might argue that distinctions between major organs and tissues are mere cultural constructions; nevertheless, this boundary is crucial to medical discourse, legislation, and constructions of personhood, in various ways, by involved parties. Corneas, pituitary glands, and heart valves, for example, are categorized as tissues (as are bones, among the oldest of human parts to be traded on the global market). Tissues are easier to harvest than major organs in a multitude of ways. . . . The removal of major organs, in contrast, requires complex bio-technical machinery, anesthetic expertise, and surgical competence if they are to remain viable" (Sharp's "Response," in Scheper-Hughes 2000, 217).

3 A situation poignantly dramatized by the death in 2004 of Christopher Reeve, the actor who played Superman in a series of films. Reeve became quadriplegic as the result of an equestrian accident. He also became a vigorous advocate for stem-cell research, involved in fund-raising and public speaking despite his need for a ventilator. He frequently expressed the belief that stem-cell research would enable him and other people with spinal injuries to walk again. He died of infection arising from pressure sores.

4 For an overview of the history of organ transplantation in the United States, see the final report of the task force authorized by the National Organ Transplant Act (U.S. Task Force on Organ Transplantation 1986, 15–19). Amendments to the Social Security Act enacted in 1972 were tremendously important for kidney transplants. As Laura G. Dooley and Robert S. Gaston note, in that year Congress "grant[ed] patients with irreversible kidney failure the right to government-subsidized, long term care in the form of either dialysis or transplantation." This action legally committed the federal government to play a key mediating role in kidney transplantation, and effectively committed it to a similar role regarding other forms of organ transplantation (Dooley and Gaston 1998, 704, see also 709).

5 This "act" was not a piece of legislation but rather a recommendation from the National Conference of Commissioners on Uniform State Laws (NCCUSL), an "organization [that] comprises more than 300 lawyers, judges and law professors, appointed by the states as well as the District of Columbia, Puerto Rico and the U.S. Virgin Islands, to draft proposals for uniform and model laws on subjects where uniformity is desirable and practicable, and work toward their enactment in legislatures" (http://www.nccusl.org/nccusl/DesktopDefault.aspx; accessed 4 December 2004). The UAGA of 1968 was subsequently adopted by all fifty states and the District of Columbia.

6 Harrison has argued that organs such as kidneys were "gifts" in the 1970s in large part because the lack of effective anti-rejection drugs made it necessary to solicit kidneys from family members, who were clearly less likely to consider asking for money from another family member (Harrison 1999, 27). Barnett and Kaserman make the same claim, though as we outline below, they position this as a "historical accident" in order to argue against the gift system itself (Barnett and Kaserman 2000, 342–43).

7 As Susan C. Lawrence notes, "[t]he various 'anatomical' and 'tissue' acts governing dissection and organ transplants have major loopholes . . . when it comes to the disposition of human material not for therapeutic purposes, but for medical and scientific research. The 1987 amended Uniform Anatomical Gift act (which most states have adopted in some form or other), for example, prohibits the sale of organs and tissues for transplant, but *not*—by obvious omission—for use in teaching and research" (Lawrence 1998, 122).

8 In 1991 the journalist Peter Young outlined the specific costs charged by the Oklahoma Organ Sharing Network for organ "acquisition" in the case of Susan Renea Sutton, who had committed suicide. He noted that "at least $22,000" went to the Oklahoma nonprofit, a fee that "included $460 for each of four ambulance trips (pick up and delivery of the heart and the liver); $9,000 to $10,000 for the hospital where Ms. Sutton died (covering operating room, intensive care and medications to maintain the body); $300 to $400 for blood testing to protect organ recipients against illnesses like AIDS and hepatitis; $800 for kidney type matching; and $8000 for the transplant agency's overhead, or salaries, office space and telephone" (Young 1994, § B, 7).

9 For economic critiques of the "spot" market proposal see Guttmann 1991 and Tietzel 2001. Both stress the small number of cadavers from which viable organs can be harvested; Tietzel also points out that a selling price of $1,000 might be less money than "the transaction costs of writing that contract" for the exchange (Tietzel 2001, 162).

10 For other examples of live donor market proposals see Joralemon 1995, 335–36. While fewer such proposals exist, Joralemon astutely points out that even a few of these effectively shift the "center" of debate toward market solutions, for "[o]utlandish proposals for a fully free market in bodily organs . . . mak[e] other proposals seem more moderate by comparison" (Joralemon 2001, 32).

11 Figures for 1988 from Harrison 1999, 24. Figures for 1993, 1998, and 2004 from the UNOS website (http://www.unos.org; accessed 4 December 2004).

12 Data for 1993 and 1998 from the OPTN/SRTR annual report for 2003 (http://www.optn.org/AR2003/default.htm; accessed 4 December 2004). Data for 2003 from the New York Organ Donor Network website, "Data" section (http://www.donatelifeny.org/organ/o_statistics.html; accessed 4 December 2004). It is worth noting that the historical increase in the number of people on organ transplantation waiting lists tends to be far more prominently displayed than data pertaining to the historical increase of the number of deaths of those on waiting lists. This is probably due, at least in part, to the decreasing proportion over the last decade of those who have died while on waiting lists: 8.9 percent in 1993, 8.2 percent in 1998, and 7.7 percent in 2002.

13 In the 1990s reports of kidney prices ranged from $1,000 to what John Frow suggested in 1997 was the "somewhat implausible price of $200,000" (Frow 1997, 163–66). Frow also provides a useful outline of the key "figures" and "metaphors" that have organized popular media accounts of these distribution networks (Frow 1997, 162–79).

14 See for example http://sunsite.berkeley.edu/biotech/organswatch/ ; accessed 4 December 2004.

15 Scheper-Hughes appeals to precisely the same values when she argues that "[t]he discourse on scarcity [of organs] conceals the overproduction of excess and wasted organs that daily end up in hospital dumpsters in parts of the world where the necessary transplant infrastructure is limited" and suggests that impoverished residents of third world countries ought to be the recipients of these organs (Scheper-Hughes 2000, 198).

16 The eBay policy for "Human Parts and Remains" is now as follows: "Humans, the human body or any human body parts may not be listed on eBay. Examples of prohibited items include, but are not limited to: organs, bone, blood, waste, sperm, and eggs. You may not include such items as a gift, prize or giveaway in connection with an item listed on eBay. Items that contain human hair (e.g., lockets) as well as skulls and skeletons that are used for educational purposes may be listed on eBay." See http://pages.ebay.com/help/policies/remains.html; accessed 4 December 2004. For a discussion of eBay in the context of online auctions in general see Lucking-Reiley 2000.

17 As Cohen notes, traditional antiques dealers depended upon the knowledge that information about prices would *not* flow from potential buyers to potential sellers. This is because dealers depended upon a system of "pickers": "buyers who go out to estate sales, flea markets, and country auctions, hunting down antiques," which they then purchase and sell to a dealer, who in turn sells to consumers for a large markup (Cohen 2002, 108, see also 172).

18 It is worth noting, however, that apparently serious ads from both would-be organ sellers and buyers appeared in the classified advertisement sections of newspapers in the early 1980s (Blair and Kaserman 1991, 416, citing Chapman 1984), and again on web sites such as Organs Watch in the early twenty-first century (Scheper-Hughes 2002b, 42, 51). The eBay auction differed from these previous attempts in that the escalating bids could be publicly tracked.

19 See http://pages.ebay.com/help/community/values.html; accessed 4 December 2004. From its origins eBay had sought to integrate these "community values" into its site architecture through features such as bulletin boards, chat rooms, a "Community Help Forum," workshops, a newsletter, a library of articles, online seller-rating systems, and even an "in-person" conference.

20 By 1999, the year of its kidney scandal, eBay had registered users from ninety countries and these exchanges were not, and could not be, monitored by any central agency (Cohen 2002, 187).

21 The auction form has appealed to a number of health care providers. In the late 1990s what we might call a "first wave" of auction sites attempted to establish business-to-business bidding on health care products. Pharmabid.com, for example, set up auctions for hospital supplies, including plasma and albumin. While many if not all of these sites failed relatively quickly, a second wave of health care auction services has proved more successful. Bidshift, for example, offers software for hospital staffing that allows managers to post open shifts, and employees to "dynamically bid" on those shifts by specifying availability and the desired hourly rate of pay. Bidshift seems to be doing well, and has been adopted by several regional hospital systems. See http://www.bidshift.com/html/customers.html, and for general information, http://www.bidshift.com/index.html; accessed 4 December 2004.

22 Titmuss had outlined a similar dynamic with blood, arguing that because of the increasing use of surgery in countries such as the United States, "there may be no predictable limits to future requirements for blood in high income countries" (Titmuss 1997, 81).

23 Data from http://www.unos.org; accessed 4 December 2004.

24 In 2004, of 86,883 people on all organ waiting lists in the United States, 11,559 were waiting for a "repeat transplant." In 1988 there were 38 multiple-organ transplantations conducted in the United States; in 1993, 92; in 1998, 184; in 2003, 348. Data from http://www.unos.org; accessed 4 December 2004. For discussion of the increase in conditions for which transplantation has been deemed acceptable, see Scheper-Hughes 2002b, 49–50).

25 The figures for multiple-organ transplants are even more striking: in 1988, 0.9 percent of all multiple-organ transplants in the United States went to patients over the age of sixty-five, while in 2003 the figure was 21.1 percent. Data from http://www.unos.org; accessed 4 December 2004.

Conclusion

1 Thanks to Adele Clarke for this point.

2 If we look beyond Europe and the settler populations of North America, we can also identify new spheres of negotiation opening up between indigenous peoples and biocommerce. Indigenous groups approached by researchers seeking DNA samples have developed international principles in favor of community consultation and consent, and benefit sharing of both knowledge and profits. These principles have recently been codified in the UN International Declaration on Human Genetic Data of 2004 (Kaye 2004b). It seems likely that this instrument will be used in nonindigenous contexts in the future.

Bibliography

Adams, A. F., A. H. Barnett, and D. L. Kaserman. 1999. "Markets for Organs: The Question of Supply." *Contemporary Economics Policy* 17:147–55.

Agres, T. 2003. "Coming Clean on Stem Cells." *Scientist*, 21 January. www.the-scientist.com. Accessed 24 January 2003.

Allison, R. 2002. "Doctor in Organ Sale Scandal Struck Off." *Guardian*, 31 August, 7.

American Medical Association, Working Group on Ethical Issues in Umbilical Cord Blood Banking. 1997. *Journal of the American Medical Association* 278:938–43.

Anderson, B. 1991. *Imagined Communities: Reflections on the Origin and Spread of Nationalism*. London: Verso.

Anderson, D., F. Gage, and I. Weissman. 2001. "Can Stem Cells Cross Lineage Boundaries?" *Nature Medicine* 7: 393–95.

Anderson, W. L., and A. H. Barnett. 1999. "Waiting for Transplants." *Free Market* 17:1–8.

Andrews, L., and D. Nelkin. 2001. *Body Bazaar: The Market for Human Tissue in the Biotechnology Age*. New York: Crown.

Appadurai, A. 1986. "Introduction: Commodities and the Politics of Value." *The Social Life of Things: Commodities in Cultural Perspective*, ed. A. Appadurai. Cambridge: Cambridge University Press. 3–63.

Armitage, S., et al. 1999. "Cord Blood Banking in London: The First 1000 Collections." *Bone Marrow Transplantation* 24:139–45.

Arrighi, G. 1994. *The Long Twentieth Century: Money, Power and the Origins of Our Times*. London: Verso.

Ballin, A. 1995. "Autologous Umbilical Cord Blood Transfusion." *Archives of Disease in Childhood* 73:181–83.

Barlow, J. P. 1994. "The Economy of Ideas." *Wired* 2, no. 3.

Barnett, A. H., T. R. Beard, and D. L. Kaserman. 1993. "The Medical Community's Opposition to Organ Markets: Ethics or Economics?" *Review of Industrial Organization* 8:669–78.

———. 1996. "Scope, Learning, and Cross-Subsidy: Organ Transplants in a Multi-Division Hospital: An Extension." *Southern Economic Journal* 62:760–67.

Barnett, A. H., and D. L. Kaserman. 1995. "The 'Rush to Transplant' and Organ Shortages." *Economic Inquiry* 33:506–15.

———. 2000. "Comment on 'The Shortage in Market-Inalienable Human Organs': Faulty Analysis of a Failed Policy." *American Journal of Economics and Sociology* 59:339–45.

Baslar, K. 1998. *The Concept of the Common Heritage of Mankind in International Law.* The Hague: Martinus Nijhoff.

Bayer, R. 1999. "Blood and AIDS in America: The Making of a Catastrophe." *Blood Feuds: AIDS, Blood, and the Politics of Medical Disaster,* ed. E. Feldman and R. Bayer. New York: Oxford University Press.

Beck, U. 1992. *Risk Society: Towards a New Modernity.* London: Sage.

Behrman, M., and H. Keim. 1992. "Intraoperative and Postoperative Red Blood Cell Salvage." *Contemporary Orthopaedics* 24:165–69.

Berridge, V. 1996. *AIDS in the UK: The Making of Policy, 1981–1994.* Oxford: Oxford University Press.

Bhopal, R., et al. 1992. "Perceptions about Blood Donation, Transfusion and the Risk of HIV Infection: Implications for the Blood Transfusion Service." *AIDS Care* 4:43–52.

Bizzaro, J. W. 2004. "An Open Letter to the NIH." http://bioinformatics. org/. Accessed 4 December 2004.

Blackburn, R. 2002. *Banking on Death, or, Investing in Life: The History and Future of Pensions.* New York: Verso.

Blair, R., and D. Kaserman. 1991. "The Economics and Ethics of Alternative Cadaveric Organ Procurement Policies." *Yale Journal on Regulation* 8:403–52.

Boulier, W. 1995. "Note: Sperm, Spleens, and Other Valuables: The Need to Recognize Property Rights in Human Body Parts." *Hofstra Law Review* 23:693–731.

Bourdieu, P. 1977. *Outline of a Theory of Practice.* New York: Cambridge University Press.

———. 1984. *Distinction: A Social Critique of the Judgement of Taste.* London: Routledge and Kegan Paul.

Bourque, J., and J. Sugerman. 2000. "Banking on the Future." *Forum for Applied Research and Public Policy*, spring, 65–68.

Bowcott, O. 1989. "Trade in Human Organs 'Increasing Aids Risk.'" *Guardian*, 6 December, 3.

———. 1990a. "World Scramble for Kidneys Exploits Poor: Disciplinary Hearing Sheds Light on Third World Market Which Makes Peasants and Criminals Hostages to Advances in Medical Science." *Guardian*, 5 April, 4.

———. 1990b. "Patients' Plight Moved Surgeon." *Guardian*, 5 April, 4.

Boyle, J. 1996. *Shamans, Software, and Spleens: Law and the Construction of the Information Society*. Cambridge: Harvard University Press.

———. 2003. "The Second Enclosure Movement and the Construction of the Public Domain." *Law and Contemporary Problems* 66, nos. 1–2: 33–74.

Bromley, D. W., ed. 1992. *Making the Commons Work: Theory, Practice, and Policy*. San Francisco: ICS.

Brown, S. A., et al. 2002. "The Genetic Age: Who Owns the Genome? A Symposium on Intellectual Property and the Human Genome." *John Marshall Review of Intellectual Property Law* 6:4–29.

Broxmeyer, H., et al. 1990. "Human Umbilical Cord Blood: A Clinically Useful Source of Transplantable Hematopoietic Stem/Progenitor Cells." *International Journal of Cell Cloning* 8, suppl. 1:76–89.

Broxmeyer, H., G. Douglas, G. Hangoc, et al. 1989. "Human Umbilical Cord Blood as a Potential Source of Transplantable Hematopoietic Stem/Progenitor Cells." *Procedures of the National Academy of Science USA* 86:3828–32.

Burglo, R., E. Gluckman, and F. Locatelli. 2003. "Ethical Reappraisal of 15 Years of Cord Blood Transplantation." *Lancet*, 18 January, 250–52.

Bush, G. W. 2001. "Stem Cell Science and the Preservation of Life." *New York Times*, 12 August, § 4, 13.

Butler, L. 1982. "The Commons Concept: An Historical Concept with Modern Relevance." *William and Mary Law Review* 23:835–935.

Butler, P. 2001. "How the Cities Have Responded to the Terrorist Attack." *Guardian*, 13 September.

Callon, M. 1998. "Introduction: The Embeddedness of Economic Markets in Economics." *The Laws of the Markets*, ed. M. Callon. Oxford: Blackwell.

Caplan, A. 2003. "Soldiers' Sperm Offers Biological Insurance Policy." http://Bioethics.net. Accessed 4 December 2004.

"Casualties and Donors Flood Hospitals." 2001. *Guardian*, 12 September.

Caulfield, T. 2003. "From Human Genes to Stem Cells: New Challenges for Patent Law?" *Trends in Biotechnology* 21:101–3.

Chapman, F. S. 1984. "The Life-and-Death Question of an Organ Market." *Fortune*, 11 June, 108–15.

Chase, D., et al. 1998. "The North Cumbria Community Genetics Project." *Journal of Medical Genetics* 35: 413–16.

Chief Medical Officer's Expert Group. 2000. *Stem Cell Research: Medical Progress with Responsibility: Report from the Chief Medical Officer's Expert Group Reviewing the Potential of Developments in Stem Cell Research and Cell Nuclear Replacement to Benefit Human Health*. United Kingdom, Department of Health.

Clay, M., and W. Block. 2002. "A Free Market for Human Organs." *Journal of Social, Political, and Economic Studies* 27:227–36.

Cohen, A. 2002. *The Perfect Store: Inside eBay*. New York: Little, Brown.

Cohen, L. R. 1989. "Increasing the Supply of Transplant Organs: The Virtues of a Futures Market." *George Washington Law Review* 58:1–51.

——. 2002. "The Other Kidney: Biopolitics beyond Recognition." *Commodifying Bodies*, ed. Nancy Scheper-Hughes and Loïc Wacquant. London: Sage. 9–30.

Comité Consultatif National d'Ethique. 2002. *Umbilical Cord Blood Banks for Autologous Use or for Research: Opinion No. 74*.

Cooper, M. 2006. "Resuscitations: Stem Cells and the Crisis of Old Age." *Body and Society* 12.

Corrigan, O. 2003. "Empty Ethics: The Problem with Informed Consent." *Sociology of Health and Illness* 25:768–92.

Council of Europe. 1997. Convention for the Protection of Human Rights and Dignity of the Human Being with Regard to the Application of Biology and Medicine: Convention on Human Rights and Biomedicine. Oviedo: Council of Europe.

——. 2000. "Autologous Blood Donation and Transfusion in Europe: Report of the 1997 Data." Available at http://www.social.coe.int/en/index.htm. Accessed 20 August 2003.

Crichton, M. 1990. *Jurassic Park*. New York: Alfred A. Knopf.

Dasgupta, P., and P. David. 1994. "Toward a New Economics in Science." *Research Policy* 23:487–521.

De Haan, G., et al. 2003. "In Vitro Generation of Long-Term Repopulating Hematopoietic Stem Cells by Fibroblast Growth Factor-1." *Developmental Cell* 4:241–51.

Derrida, J. 1992. *Given Time.* Vol. 1: *Counterfeit Money.* Chicago: University of Chicago Press.

Dickenson, D. 2002. "Commodification of Human Tissue: Implications for Feminist and Development Ethics." *Developing World Bioethics* 2:55–63.

Dooley, L. G., and R. S. Gaston. 1998. "Stumbling toward Equity: The Role of Government in Kidney Transplantation." *University of Illinois Law Review* 1998, no. 3:703–25.

Douglas, M. 1984. *Purity and Danger: An Analysis of the Concepts of Pollution and Taboo.* London: Routledge and Kegan Paul.

Douglas, M., and B. Isherwood. 1979. *The World of Goods: Towards an Anthropology of Consumption.* London: Routledge.

Doyle, R. 2003. *Wetwares: Experiments in Postvital Living.* Minneapolis: University of Minnesota Press.

Ecologist. 1993. *Whose Common Future? Reclaiming the Commons.* Philadelphia: New Society.

Egan, M. 2000. "Cell Makers: Biotechs ViaCell and Aastrom Harvest and Grow Stem Cells." *Forbes,* 11 December, 220–22.

Eisenberg, R. S. 1996. "Public Research and Private Development: Patents and Technology Transfer in Government-Sponsored Research." *Virginia Law Review* 82:1663–1727.

Ericson, R., D. Barry, and A. Doyle. 2000. "The Moral Hazards of Neoliberalism: Lessons from the Private Insurance Industry." *Economy and Society* 29:532–58.

Erin, C. E., and J. A. Harris. 1994. "A Monopsonistic Market." *The Social Consequences of Life and Death under High Technology Medicine,* ed. I. Robinson. Manchester: Manchester University Press. 134–57.

European Commission. 1995. "Europeans and Blood." *Eurobarometer* 41.

Fay, M. F., et al. 1990. "Medical Waste: The Growing Issues of Management and Disposal." *AORN Journal* 51:1493–1508.

Fernandez, C., et al. 2003. "Knowledge and Attitudes of Pregnant Women with Regard to Collection, Testing and Banking of Cord Blood Stem Cells." *Canadian Medical Association Journal* 168:695–98.

Fiala, C. 2000. "No Evidence for Heterosexual HIV Transmission outside Risk Groups or Success for Prevention Campaigns." www.aliveandwell.org. Accessed 20 November 2003.

Finkel, M. 2001. "Complications." *New York Times Magazine,* 27 May, 26–33, 40, 52, 59.

Finucane, M., P. Slovic, and C. Mertz. 2000. "Public Perception of the Risk of Blood Transfusion." *Transfusion* 40:1017–22.

Fontaine, P. 2002. "Blood, Politics and Social Science: Richard Titmuss and the Institute of Economic Affairs, 1957–1973." *Isis* 93:401–34.

Forgie, M., et al. 1998. "Pre-operative Autologous Donation Decreases Allogenic Transfusion but Increases Exposure to All Red Cell Transfusion." *Archives of Internal Medicine* 58:610–16.

Foucault, M. 1980. *The History of Sexuality*. Vol. 1: *An Introduction*, trans. Robert Hurley. New York: Vintage.

——. 1984. "What Is an Author?" *The Foucault Reader*, ed. P. Rabinow. New York: Pantheon.

Fox, R. C., and J. P. Swazey. 1992. *Spare Parts: Organ Replacement in American Society*. New York: Oxford University Press.

Franceschi, S., L. Dal Maso, and C. La Vecchia. 1995. "Trends in Incidence of AIDS Associated with Transfusion of Blood and Blood Products in Europe and the United States, 1985–93." *British Medical Journal* 311:1534–36.

Fredrickson, J. 1998. "Comment: Umbilical Cord Blood Stem Cells: My Body Makes Them, but Do I Get to Keep Them? Analysis of the FDA Proposed Regulations and the Impact on Individual Constitutional Property Rights." *Journal of Contemporary Health Law and Policy* 14:477–502.

Friedlaender, M. M. 2002. "The Right to Sell or Buy a Kidney: Are We Failing Our Patients?" *Lancet* 359:971–73.

Frow, J. 1997. *Time and Commodity Culture: Essays in Cultural Theory and Postmodernity*. Oxford: Clarendon.

——. 2003. "Invidious Distinctions: Waste, Difference, and Classy Stuff." *Culture and Waste: The Creation and Destruction of Value*, ed. G. Hawkins and S. Muecke. Lanham, Md.: Rowman and Littlefield. 25–38.

Gasché, R. 1997. "Heliocentric Exchange." *The Logic of the Gift: Toward an Ethic of Generosity*, ed. A. D. Schrift. New York: Routledge.

Gershanik, J., G. Brooks, and J. Little. 1974. "Fetal Blood Lead Values in a Rural Area." *Journal of Pediatrics* 84:112–13.

Gluckman, E., H. Broxmeyer, A. Auerbach, et al. 1989. "Hematopoietic Reconstitution in a Patient with Fanconi's Anaemia by Means of Umbilical Cord Blood from an HLA-Identical Sibling." *New England Journal of Medicine* 321:1174–78.

Gold, E. R. 1996. *Body Parts: Property Rights and the Ownership of Human Biological Materials*. Washington: Georgetown University Press.

Gottlieb, K. 1998. "Human Biological Samples and the Law of Property: The Trust as a Model for Biological Repositories." *Stored Tissue Samples: Ethical, Legal and Public Policy Implications*, ed. R. Weir. Iowa City: University of Iowa Press. 182–97.

Gottweis, H. 2002. "Stem Cell Policies in the United States and in Germany: Between Bioethics and Regulation." *Policy Studies Journal* 30:444–69.

Graham, I., et al. 1999. "Autologous versus Allogenic Transfusion: Patients' Perceptions and Experiences." *Canadian Medical Association Journal* 160:989–95.

Guttmann, R. 1991. "The Meaning of 'The Economics and Ethics of Alternative Cadaveric Organ Procurement Policies.'" *Yale Journal on Regulation* 8:453–62.

Habermas, J. 2003. *The Future of Human Nature.* Cambridge: Polity.

Hardin, G. 1968. "The Tragedy of the Commons." *Science* 162:1243–48.

Harman, A. 1999. "Auction for a Kidney Pops Up on Ebay's Site." *New York Times*, 3 September, § A, 13.

Harrell, G. P., and C. Catanzariti. 1994. "Federal and State Regulation of Medical Waste." *Journal of Legal Medicine* 15:1–88.

Harris, J., and C. Erin. 2002. "An Ethically Defensible Market in Organs." *British Medical Journal* 325:114–15.

Harrison, T. 1999. "Globalization and the Trade in Human Body Parts." *Canadian Review of Sociology and Anthropology* 36:21–35.

Harry, D. 1995. "Patenting of Life and Its Implications for Indigenous People." Available at http://www.ipcb.org/publications/briefing_papers/files/patents.html. Accessed 25 October 2004.

Hawkins, G., and S. Muecke. 2003. "Introduction: Cultural Economies of Waste." *Culture and Waste: The Creation and Destruction of Value*, ed. G. Hawkins and S. Muecke. Lanham, Md.: Rowman and Littlefield. ix–xvii.

Hayden, C. P. 1998. "A Biodiversity Sampler for the Millennium." *Reproducing Reproduction: Kinship, Power, and Technological Innovation*, ed. S. Franklin and H. Ragoné. Philadelphia: University of Pennsylvania Press.

———. 2003. *When Nature Goes Public: The Making and Unmaking of Bioprospecting in Mexico.* Princeton: Princeton University Press.

Healy, K. 1999. "The Emergence of HIV in the U.S. Blood Supply: Organizations, Obligations, and the Management of Uncertainty." *Theory and Society* 28: 529–58.

Hiatt, H. H. 1975. "Protecting the Medical Commons: Who Is Responsible?" *New England Journal of Medicine* 293:235–41.

Hirschler, Ben. 2003. "Stem Cells May Eliminate Need for Heart Transplant." www.reuters.com. Accessed 9 March 2003.

Hogle, L. F. 1999. *Recovering the Nation's Body: Cultural Memory, Medi-*

cine, and the Politics of Redemption. New Brunswick: Rutgers University Press.

———. 2003. "Life/Time Warranty: Rechargeable Cells and Extendable Lives." *Remaking Life and Death: Toward an Anthropology of the Biosciences*, ed. S. Franklin and M. Lock. Santa Fe: School of American Research Press. 61–96.

———. 2004. "Engraftment Strategies: Relations of Policy-Making and Research in Stem Cell Biology." 4S/EASST Conference, 25–29 August, École des Mines, Paris.

Holden, C. 1993. "Banking a Cord Earns Interest." *Science* 262:1511.

House of Lords. 2002. Report from the Select Committee on Stem Cell Research, 27 February. HL 83(i).

Hughes, C. 1991. "Egypt's Desperate Trade: Body Parts for Sale." *New York Times*, 23 September, § A, 1, 8.

Human Fertilisation and Embryology Authority. 2001. *Code of Practice*, 5th edn. London.

Human Genetics Advisory Commission. 1998. *Cloning Issues in Reproduction, Science and Medicine*.

Hurley, R. 1995. *Human Tissue: Ethical and Legal Issues*. London: Nuffield Council on Bioethics.

Jana, M. 2003. "Cord Blood Controversy." *Newsweek*, 18 August, 56–57.

Joralemon, D. 1995. "Organ Wars: The Battle for Body Parts." *Medical Anthropology Quarterly* 9:335–56.

———. 2000. "The Ethics of the Organ Market: Lloyd R. Cohen and the Free Marketeers." *Biotechnology and Culture: Bodies, Anxieties, Ethics*, ed. P. E. Brodwin. Indianapolis: Indiana University Press. 224–37.

———. 2001. "Shifting Ethics: Debating the Incentive Question in Organ Transplantation." *Journal of Medical Ethics* 27:30–35.

Joyner, C. C. 2001. "Global Commons: The Oceans, Antarctica, the Atmosphere, and Outer Space." *Managing Global Issues: Lessons Learned*, ed. P. J. Simmons and C. de Jonge Oudrat. Washington: Carnegie Endowment for International Peace. 354–91.

Kaldor, M. 1999. *New and Old Wars: Organized Violence in a Global Era*. Cambridge: Polity.

Kant, I. 1981 [1785]. *Grounding for a Metaphysics of Morals*, trans. James Ellington. Indianapolis: Hackett.

Kaye, J. 2004a. "Abandoning Informed Consent: The Case of Genetic Research in Population Collections." *The Gift: The Donation and Exploi-*

tation of Human Tissue in Genetic Research, ed. R. Tutton and O. Corrigan. London: Routledge.

——. 2004b. "Indigenous Influences: Tracing These Principles in the Population Genetics Debate." Paper presented at the 7th World Congress of Bioethics, University of New South Wales, Sydney, 9–12 November.

Kelmenson, L.-A. 1979. "Whatever Happened to U. S. Innovation?" *New York Times*, 4 February, § F, 14.

Kimbrell, A. 1993. *The Human Body Shop: The Engineering and Marketing of Life*. San Francisco: Harper Collins.

——. 1997. *The Human Body Shop: The Cloning, Engineering, and Marketing of Life*. 2d edn. Washington: Gateway.

Kline, R. 2001. "Whose Blood Is It, Anyway?" *Scientific American* 284:42–49.

Knowles, S., and S. Adams. 2001–2. "Bioethics Symposium: Who Owns My DNA? The National and International Intellectual Property Laws on Human Embryonic Tissue and Cloning." *Cumberland Law Review* 32:457.

Knudtzin, S. 1974. "In Vitro Growth of Granulocytic Colonies from Circulating Cells in Human Cord Blood." *Blood* 43:357–61.

Kopytoff, I. 1986. "The Cultural Biography of Things." *The Social Life of Things: Commodities in Cultural Perspective*, ed. A. Appadurai. Cambridge: Cambridge University Press.

Korner, D., L. Rosenberg, M. Aledort, et al. 1994. "HIV-1 Infection Incidence among Persons with Hemophilia in the United States and Western Europe, 1978–1990." *Journal of Acquired Immunodeficiency Syndrome* 7:279–86.

Kristeva, J. 1982. *Powers of Horror: An Essay on Abjection*, trans. L. Roudiez. New York: Columbia University Press.

Landecker, H. 2000. "Immortality, in Vitro: A History of the HeLa Cell Line." *Biotechnology and Culture: Bodies, Anxieties, Ethics*, ed. P. E. Brodwin. Indianapolis: Indiana University Press. 53–72.

Latour, B. 1988. *The Pasteurization of France*, trans. A. Sheridan and J. Law. Cambridge: Harvard University Press.

Laughlin, M., J. Barker, B. Bambach, et al. 2001. "Hematopoietic Engraftment and Survival in Adult Recipients of Umbilical Cord Blood from Unrelated Donors." *New England Journal of Medicine* 344:1815–22.

Laurie, G. 2001. "Gift and the Paradox of the Property Paradigm." Paper presented at the seminar "Revisiting Concepts of Gift in the New Genetics," Department of Sociology, Lancaster University.

Lawrence, S. C. 1998. "Beyond the Grave: The Use and Meaning of Human Body Parts: A Historical Introduction." *Stored Tissue Samples: Ethical, Legal and Public Policy Implications*, ed. R. Weir. Iowa City: University of Iowa Press. 111–42.

Lee, B., and E. LiPuma. 2002. "Cultures of Circulation: The Imaginations of Modernity." *Public Culture* 14:191–213.

Legge, A. 2000. "Hospital Criticised for Not Obtaining Proper Consent." *British Medical Journal* 320:1291.

Lerner, J., and J. Tirole. 2002. "Some Simple Economics of Open Source." *Journal of Industrial Economics* 50:197–234.

Lessig, L. 1998. "The Architecture of Innovation." *Duke Law Journal* 51:1783–1801.

———. 2001. *The Future of Ideas: The Fate of the Commons in a Connected World*. New York: Random House.

Litman, J. 1990. "The Public Domain." *Emory Law Journal* 39:965–1009.

Lock, M. 2001. "The Alienation of Body Tissue and the Biopolitics of Immortalized Cell Lines." *Body and Society* 7:63–91.

———. 2002. *Twice Dead: Organ Transplants and the Reinvention of Death*. Berkeley: University of California Press.

Locke, J. 1988. *Two Treatises on Government*. Cambridge: Cambridge University Press.

Lockwood, C. 2002. "Should We Encourage Storage of Umbilical Cord Stem Cells?" *Contemporary Obstetrics/Gynecology*, November. 8–9.

Lucking-Reiley, D. 2000. "Auctions on the Internet: What's Being Auctioned, and How?" *Journal of Industrial Economics* 48:227–52.

Lupton, D. 1997. "Consumerism, Reflexivity and the Medical Encounter." *Social Science and Medicine* 45:373–81.

MacAskill, S., et al. 1989. "Scottish Attitudes to Blood Donation and AIDS." *British Medical Journal* 298:1012–14.

Mackay-Sim, A. 2004. "Adult Stem Cells from the Olfactory Epithelium: A Potential Source of Autologous Therapies." Paper presented at the 4th NSW Stem Cell Network Workshop, 16 March, Prince of Wales Hospital, Sydney.

Manns, Leslie D. 1995. "Regulation of On-Site Medical Waste Incinerators in the United States and the United Kingdom: Is the Public Interest Being Served?" *Journal of Economic Issues* 29:545–54.

Martlew, V. 1997. "Transfusion Medicine towards the Millennium." R.

Titmuss, *The Gift Relationship: From Human Blood to Social Policy*, ed. A. Oakley and J. Ashton. London: LSE. 41–54.

Marx, K., and F. Engels. 1978. *The Marx-Engels Reader*, ed. R. C. Tucker. New York: W. W. Norton.

Maskus, K. E. 2000. *Intellectual Property Rights in the Global Economy*. Washington: Institute for International Economics.

Maskus, K. E., and J. H. Reichman. 2003. "International Public Goods and Transfer of Technology under a Globalized Intellectual Property Regime." Published draft of a paper for the Conference on International Public Goods and Transfer of Technology Under a Globalized Intellectual Property Regime, Duke University, 4–6 April, 1–20.

Maurer, S. M., A. Rai, and A. Sali. 2004. "Finding Cures for Tropical Diseases: Is Open Source an Answer?" *PLoS Medicine* 1:e56.

Mauss, M. 1990 [1950]. *The Gift: The Form and Reason for Exchange in Archaic Societies*, trans. W. Halls. London: Routledge.

McCormack, S., and R. Cook-Deegan. 1999. "DNA Patent Database." Available at http://dnapatents.georgetown.edu.

McElheny, V. K. 1976. "An Industrial 'Innovation Crisis' Is Decried at M.I.T. Symposium." *New York Times*, 10 December, 85.

McLaren, A. 2000. "Cloning: Pathways to a Pluripotent Future." *Science* 288: 1775–80.

McNally, R., and P. Wheale. 1998. "The Consequences of Modern Genetic Engineering: Patents, 'Nomads' and the 'Bio-Industrial Complex.'" *The Social Management of Genetic Engineering*, ed. P. Wheale, R. von Schomberg, and P. Glasner. Aldershot: Ashgate. 303–30.

Medical Research Council. 2001. *Human Tissue and Biological Samples for Use in Research: Operational and Ethical Guidelines*. MRC Ethics Series, April.

Meek, J., and P. Brown. 2000. "Patenting Life: How US Muscle Bent the Rules in Europe." *Guardian*, 15 November.

Mitchell, R. 2004. "$ell: Body Wastes, Information and Commodification." *Data Made Flesh: Embodying Information*, ed. R. Mitchell and P. Thurtle. New York: Routledge. 121–36.

Mitchell, W. J. T. 1998. *The Last Dinosaur Book: The Life and Times of a Cultural Icon*. Chicago: University of Chicago Press.

Moore v. Regents of the University of California. 1988. 215 Cal. App. 3d 709, 249 Cal. Rptr. 494.

Moore v. Regents of the University of California. 1990. 51 Cal. 3d 120, 793 P.2d 479, 271 Cal. Rptr. 146.

Moser, W. 2002. "The Acculturation of Waste." *Waste-Site Stories: The*

Recycling of Memory, ed. B. Neville and J. Villeneuve. Albany: State University of New York Press.

Mowery, D. C., et al. 2004. *Ivory Tower and Industrial Innovation: University-Industry Technology Transfer before and after the Bayh-Dole Act in the United States.* Stanford: Stanford Business Books.

Mulkay, M. 1997. *The Embryo Research Debate: Science and the Politics of Reproduction.* Cambridge: Cambridge University Press.

Munzer, S. 1994. "An Uneasy Case against Property Rights in Body Parts." *Social Philosophy and Policy* 11:259–86.

Mustonen, M. 2003. "Copyleft: The Economics of Linux and Other Open Source Software." *Information Economics and Policy* 15:99–121.

Nagai, M. 1998. "History of Autologous Blood Transfusion in Neurosurgical Operations." *Neurological Surgery* 26:1117–22.

Naser, C. 1998. "Researcher Obligations to Tissue and DNA Sample Sources." *Stored Tissue Samples: Ethical, Legal and Public Policy Implications*, ed. R. Weir. Iowa City: University of Iowa Press. 160–81.

National Blood Service. 2002. *Working Together to Deliver Improvements: Annual Report 2002.* United Kingdom, National Health Service.

Nau, J. 1993. "Placental Albumin." *Lancet* 342:1479.

Neilson, B. 2003. "Globalization and the Biopolitics of Aging." *CR: The New Centennial Review* 3:161–86.

Noel, L. 1999. "The Impact of HIV in France." *Transfusion Medicine* 9:351–82.

Novas, C., and N. Rose. 2000. "Genetic Risk and the Birth of the Somatic Individual." *Economy and Society* 29:485–513.

Nutbeam, D., et al. 1989. "Public Knowledge and Attitudes to AIDS." *Public Health* 103:205–11.

Oakley, A., and J. Ashton. 1997. "Introduction to the New Edition." R. Titmuss, *The Gift Relationship: From Human Blood to Social Policy*, ed. A. Oakley and J. Ashton. London: LSE.

Ostrom, E. 1990. *Governing the Commons: The Evolution of Institutions for Collective Action.* Cambridge: Cambridge University Press.

Palsson, G., and P. Rabinow. 2001. "The Icelandic Genome Debate." *Trends in Biotechnology* 19:166–71.

Parry, G. 1990a. "Struck-off Specialist Defends Kidney Sale." *Guardian*, 5 April, 1.

———. 1990b. "Farmer Fell Prey to Organ Harvesters." *Guardian*, 5 April, 4.

———. 1990c. " 'Broker' Accuses Other Doctors." *Guardian*, 5 April, 4.

———. 1990d. "Specialist Who Made Success His Business." *Guardian*, 5 April, 4.

"Patent Bill Seeks Shift to Bolster Innovation." 1979. *Washington Post*, 8 April, ¶ M, 1.

People Science and Policy. 2003. *Public Consultation on the Stem Cell Bank: Report Prepared for the Medical Research Council*. London: People Science and Policy.

Peters, T. 1991. "Life or Death: The Issue of Payment in Cadaveric Organ Donation." *Journal of the American Medical Association* 265:1302–5.

Pixley, J. 2004. *Emotions in Finance: Distrust and Uncertainty in Global Markets*. Cambridge: Cambridge University Press.

Politis, C., and C. Richardson. 2001. "Autologous Blood Donation and Transfusion in Europe." *Vox Sanguinis* 81:119–23.

Pottage, A. 1998. "The Inscription of Life in Law: Genes, Patents and Biopolitics." *Modern Law Review* 61:740–65.

Rabinow, P. 1996. *Essays on the Anthropology of Reason*. Princeton: Princeton University Press.

———. 1999. *French DNA: Trouble in Purgatory*. Chicago: University of Chicago Press.

Radcliffe-Richards, J., et al. 1998. "The Case for Allowing Kidney Sales." *Lancet* 351:1950–52.

Raghunathan, A. 2001. "Umbilical Cord Blood May Be Biological Insurance." *Times Herald-Record*, 9 December.

Rensberger, B. 1972. "Technology Lag Stirs Scientists." *New York Times*, 20 July, 29.

Reubinoff, B., et al. 2001. "Neural Progenitors from Human Embryonic Stem Cells." *Nature Biotechnology* 19:1134–40.

Robertson, B., and D. McQueen. 1994. "Perceived Risk of Becoming Infected with HIV by Donating Blood and Changes in Reported Blood Donation Practice among the Scottish General Public, 1989–1992." *AIDS Care* 6:435–42.

Rose, C. 1986. "The Comedy of the Commons: Custom, Commerce, and Inherently Public Property." *University of Chicago Law Review* 53:711–81.

Rose, N., and C. Novas. 2004. "Biological Citizenship." *Global Assemblages: Technology, Politics, and Ethics as Anthropological Problems*, ed. A. Ong and S. Collier. Oxford: Blackwell.

Rosengarten, M. 2001. "A Pig's Tale: Porcine Viruses and Species Boundaries." *Contagion: Historical and Cultural Studies*, ed. A. Bashford and C. Hooker. London: Routledge.

Royal College of Obstetricians and Gynaecologists. 2001. *Umbilical Cord Blood Banking*. Scientific Advisory Committee Opinion Paper 2.

Royal Liverpool Children's Inquiry. 2001. *The Report of the Royal Liverpool Children's Inquiry.* Available at www.rlcinquiry.org.uk.

Rutala, W. A., R. L. Odette, and G. P. Samsa. 1989. "Management of Infectious Waste by US Hospitals." *Journal of the American Medical Association* 2622:1635–40.

Salter, B., and M. Jones. 2002. "Human Genetic Technologies, European Governance and the Politics of Bioethics." *Nature Reviews Genetics* 3:6–12.

Samuelson, P. 2001. "Digital Information, Digital Networks, and the Public Domain." Framing Papers for Duke University Conference on the Public Domain, 9–11 November. Available at http://www.law.duke.edu/pd/papers.html. 80–107.

Saywell, T. 2003. "Banking on a Chance at Life." *Far Eastern Economic Review* 166:32–34.

Schachter, O. 1983. "Comment: Human Dignity as a Normative Concept." *American Journal of International Law* 77:848–54.

Scheper-Hughes, N. 2000. "The Global Traffic in Human Organs." *Current Anthropology* 41:191–224.

———. 2002a. "Bodies for Sale: Whole or in Parts." *Commodifying Bodies*, ed. N. Scheper-Hughes and L. Wacquant. London: Sage. 1–8.

———. 2002b. "Commodity Fetishism in Organs Trafficking." *Commodifying Bodies*, ed. N. Scheper-Hughes and L. Wacquant. London: Sage. 31–62.

Schmeck, H. W., Jr. 1976. "Technology Pace Found Declining." *New York Times*, 20 April, 12.

Schmidt, P. 2002. "Blood and Disaster: Supply and Demand." *New England Journal of Medicine* 346:617–20.

Schulz, T., et al. 2003. "Directed Neuronal Differentiation of Human Embryonic Stem Cells." *BMC Neuroscience* 4:27.

Schwindt, R., and A. R. Vining. 1986. "Proposal for a Future Delivery Market for Transplant Organs." *Journal of Health Policy and Law* 11:483–500.

Sealing, K. 2002. "Great Property Cases: Teaching Fundamental Learning Techniques with *Moore v. Regents of the University of California.*" *Saint Louis University Law Journal* 46:755–74.

Shilts, R. 1987. *And the Band Played On: Politics, People and the AIDS Epidemic.* Harmondsworth: Penguin.

Shiva, V. 1997. *Biopiracy: The Plunder of Nature and Knowledge.* Boston: South End.

Shiva, V., et al. 1997. *The Enclosure and Recovery of the Commons: Biodiver-*

sity, *Indigenous Knowledge and Intellectual Property Rights.* New Delhi: Research Foundation for Science, Technology and Ecology.

Sirchia, G., and P. Rebella. 1999. "Placental/Umbilical Cord Blood Transplantation." *Haematologica* 84:738–47.

Snyder, E., and A. Vescovi. 2000. "The Possibilities/Perplexities of Stem Cells." *Nature Biotechnology* 18:827–28.

Sperling, S. 2004. "From Crisis to Potentiality: Managing Potential Selves: Stem Cells, Immigrants, and German Identity." *Science and Public Policy* 31:139–49.

Squier, S. 2000. "Life and Death at Strangeways: The Tissue-Culture Point of View." *Biotechnology and Culture: Bodies, Anxieties, Ethics,* ed. P. E. Brodwin. Indianapolis: Indiana University Press. 27–52.

Stafford, M. 1999. "Interview with Renée Fox." *Being Human: The Technological Extensions of the Body,* ed. J. Houis, P. Mieli, and M. Stafford. New York: Marsilio. 242–56.

Starr, D. 1998. *Blood: An Epic History of Medicine and Commerce.* New York: Alfred A. Knopf.

———. 2001. "Medicine, Money, and Myth: An Epic History of Blood." *Transfusion Medicine* 11:119–21.

Steering Committee of the UK Stem Cell Bank. 2004. *Code of Practice for the Use of Human Stem Cell Lines.* London: Medical Research Council.

Stevens, A. J. 2004. "The Enactment of Bayh–Dole." *Journal of Technology Transfer* 29:93–99.

Stone, A. 1996. *The Strange Case of John Moore and the Splendid Stolen Spleen: A Case Study on Science, Technology, and American Courts.* Available at http://socrates.berkeley.edu/7Eastone/research.html. Accessed 7 October 2004.

Strasser, S. 1999. *Waste and Want: A Social History of Trash.* New York: Metropolitan.

Strathern, M. 1988. *The Gender of the Gift: Problems with Women and Problems with Society in Melanesia.* Berkeley: University of California Press.

———. 1999. *Property, Substance and Effect: Anthropological Essays on Persons and Things.* London: Athlone.

Sullivan, M., et al. 2002. "Blood Collection and Transfusion in the United States in 1997." *Transfusion* 42:1253.

Sullivan, W. 1976. "Loss of Innovation in Technology Is Debated." *New York Times,* 25 November, 44.

Takacs, D. 1996. *The Idea of Biodiversity: Philosophies of Paradise.* Baltimore: Johns Hopkins University Press.

Thacker, E. 2004. *Biomedia.* Minneapolis: University of Minnesota Press.

Thompson, C. 1995. "Umbilical Cords: Turning Garbage into Clinical Gold." *Science* 268:805–6.

Thompson, M. 1979. *Rubbish Theory: The Creation and Destruction of Value.* Oxford: Oxford University Press.

Thomson, J. A., et al. 1998. "Embryonic Stem Cell Lines Derived from Human Blastocysts." *Science* 282:1145–47.

Throsby, K. 2002a. "Negotiating 'Normality' When IVF Fails." *Narrative Inquiry* 12:43–65.

——. 2002b. " 'Vials, Ampoules and a Bucketful of Syringes': The Experience of the Self-Administration of Hormonal Drugs in IVF." *Feminist Review* 72:62–77.

——. 2004. *When IVF Fails: Feminism, Infertility and the Negotiation of Normality.* London: Palgrave.

Tietzel, M. 2001. "In Praise of the Commons: Another Case Study." *European Journal of Law and Economics* 12:159–71.

Titmuss, R. 1997 [1971]. *The Gift Relationship: From Human Blood to Social Policy,* ed. A. Oakley and J. Ashton. London: LSE.

Treloar, C., et al. 2001. "Factors Influencing the Uptake of Technologies to Minimise Perioperative Allogeneic Blood Transfusion: An Interview Study of National and Institutional Stakeholders." *Internal Medicine Journal* 31:230–36.

United Kingdom, Department of Health. 2002. *Better Blood Transfusion: Appropriate Use of Blood* (Health Service circular).

U.S. Congress. 1964. *Blood Banks and Antitrust Laws: Hearings before the Subcommittee on Antitrust and Monopoly of the Committee on the Judiciary, United States Senate, Eighty-eighth Congress, Second Session, Pursuant to S. Res. 262, on S. 2560, August 18, 19, and 20, 1964.* Washington: U.S. Government Printing Office.

——. 1976. *Government Patent Policy: The Ownership of Inventions Resulting from Federal Funded Research Development: Hearings before the Subcommittee on Domestic and International Scientific Planning and Analysis of the Committee on Science and Technology, U.S. House of Representatives, Ninety-fourth Congress, Second Session, September 23, 27, 28, 29; October 1, 1976.* Washington: U.S. Government Printing Office.

——. 1978a. *Government Patent Policies: Institutional Patent Agreements: Hearings before the Subcommittee on Monopoly and Anticompetitive Activities of the Select Committee on Small Business, United States Senate, Ninety-fifth Congress, Second Session, Part I, May 22, 23, June 20, 21 and 26, 1978.* Washington: U.S. Government Printing Office.

——. 1978b. *Government Patent Policies: Institutional Patent Agreements:*

Hearings before the Subcommittee on Monopoly and Anticompetitive Activities of the Select Committee on Small Business, United States Senate, Ninety-fifth Congress, Second Session, Part 2: Appendix, May 22, 23, June 20, 21 and 26, 1978. Washington: U.S. Government Printing Office.

——. 1980a. *Patent Policy: Joint Hearing before the Committee on Commerce, Science, and Transportation and the Committee on the Judiciary, United States Senate, Ninety-sixth Congress, Second Session on Government Patent Policy, January 25, 1980.* Washington: U.S. Government Printing Office.

——. 1980b. *Government Patent Policy Act of 1980: Hearing before the Subcommittee on Science, Research, and Technology of the Committee on Science and Technology of the U.S. House of Representatives, Ninety-sixth Congress, Second Session, February 8, 1980.* Washington: U.S. Government Printing Office.

——. 1984a. *National Organ Transplant Act: Hearings before the Subcommittee on Health and the Environment of the Committee on Energy and Commerce, House of Representatives, Ninety-Eighth Congress, First Session, on H.R. 4080, July 29, October 17 and 31, 1983.* Washington: U.S. Government Printing Office.

——. 1984b. *National Organ Transplant Act: Hearing before the Subcommittee on Health of the Committee on Ways and Means, House of Representatives, Ninety-Eighth Congress, Second Session, on H.R. 4080, February 9, 1984.* Washington: U.S. Government Printing Office.

U.S. Congress, Office of Technology Assessment. 1987. *New Developments in Biotechnology: Ownership of Human Tissues and Cells: Special Report,* OTA-BA-337. Washington: U.S. Government Printing Office.

U.S. Senate. 1964. *Blood Banks and Antitrust Laws: Hearings before the Subcommittee on Antitrust and Monopoly of the Committee on the Judiciary.* Washington: U.S. Government Printing Office.

U.S. Task Force on Organ Transplantation. 1986. *Organ Transplantation: Issues and Recommendations: Report of the Task Force on Organ Transplantation.* Rockville, Md.: U.S. Department of Health and Human Services.

Urry, J. 2000. *Sociology beyond Societies: Mobilities for the Twenty-first Century.* London: Routledge.

Vastag, B. 2003. "Gene Chips Inch toward the Clinic." *Journal of the American Medical Association* 289:155–59.

Vawter, D. 1998. "An Ethical and Policy Framework for the Collection of Umbilical Cord Blood Stem Cells." *Stored Tissue Samples: Ethical,*

Legal and Public Policy Implications, ed. R. Weir. Iowa City: University of Iowa Press.

Venner v. State of Maryland. 1976. 30 Md. App. 599, 354 A.2d 483.

Vogel, G. 2002. "Pioneering Stem Cell Bank Will Soon Be Open for Deposits." *Science* 297:1784.

———. 2004. "Human Cloning: Scientists Take Step toward Therapeutic Cloning." *Science* 303:937–39.

Wald, P. 2005. "What's in a Cell? John Moore's Spleen and the Language of Bioslavery." *New Literary History* 36:205–25.

Waldby, C. 1996. *AIDS and the Body Politic: Biomedicine and Sexual Difference.* London: Routledge.

———. 2000. *The Visible Human Project: Informatic Bodies and Posthuman Medicine.* London: Routledge.

———. 2002a. "Stem Cells, Tissue Cultures and the Production of Biovalue." *Health: An Interdisciplinary Journal for the Social Study of Health, Illness and Medicine* 6:305–23.

———. 2002b. "Biomedicine, Tissue Transfer and Intercorporeality." *Feminist Theory* 3:235–50.

Waldby, C., et al. 2004. "Blood and Bioidentity: Ideas about Self, Boundaries and Risk among Blood Donors and People Living with Hepatitis C." *Social Science and Medicine* 59:1461–71.

Waldby, C., and S. Squier. 2003. "Ontogeny, Ontology and Phylogeny: Embryonic Life and Stem Cell Technologies." *Configurations: A Journal of Literature and Science* 11:27–46.

Wallace, E., et al. 1995. "Collection and Transfusion of Blood and Blood Components in the United States, 1992." *Transfusion* 35:802.

Wallace, E., et al. 1998. "Collection and Transfusion of Blood and Blood Components in the United States, 1994." *Transfusion* 38:625.

Warwick, R., and D. Fehily. n.d. "The Role of the Blood Transfusion Service in Cord Blood Banking." Available at www.health.fgov.be. Accessed 3 December 2003.

Weiner, A. B. 1992. *Inalienable Possessions: The Paradox of Keeping-While-Giving.* Berkeley: University of California Press.

Weiss, G. 1999. *Body Images: Embodiment as Intercorporeality.* London: Routledge.

World Health Organization. 2003. "Human Organ and Tissue Transplantation." Report by the Secretariat. Available at http://www.who.int/gb/ebwha.

Yelling, A. 1977. *Common Field and Enclosure in England, 1450–1850*. Hamden, Conn.: Archon.

Young, P. S. 1994. "Moving to Compensate Families in Human-Organ Market." *New York Times*, 8 July, § B, 7.

Zeitlyn, D. 2003. "Gift Economies in the Development of Open Source Software: Anthropological Reflections." *Research Policy* 32:1287–91.

Index

CATHERINE WALDBY

is a senior lecturer in medical sociology

at the University of New South Wales.

ROBERT MITCHELL

is an assistant professor of English

at Duke University.

Library of Congress Cataloging-in-Publication Data

Waldby, Cathy.
Tissue economies : blood, organs, and cell lines in late
capitalism / Catherine Waldby and Robert Mitchell.
p. ; cm. — (Science and cultural theory)
Includes bibliographical references and index.
ISBN 0-8223-3757-6 (cloth : alk. paper)
ISBN 0-8223-3770-3 (pbk. : alk. paper)
1. Tissue banks—Economic aspects. 2. Tissue banks—
Political aspects. 3. Tissue banks—Moral and ethical aspects. 4. Preservation of organs, tissues, etc.—Economic
aspects. 5. Preservation of organs, tissues, etc.—Political
aspects. 6. Preservation of organs, tissues, etc.—Moral and
ethical aspects.
[DNLM: 1. Tissue Donors—psychology—Great Britain.
2. Tissue Donors—psychology—United States. 3. Altruism—Great Britain. 4. Altruism—United States. 5. Capitalism—Great Britain. 6. Capitalism—United States. 7.
Cross-Cultural Comparison—Great Britain. 8. Cross-
Cultural Comparison—United States. 9. Social Responsibility—Great Britain. 10. Social Responsibility—United
States. 11. Tissue and Organ Procurement—economics—
Great Britain. 12. Tissue and Organ Procurement—economics—United States. 13. Tissue and Organ Procurement—organization & administration—Great Britain. 14.
Tissue and Organ Procurement—organization & admin-
istration—United States. QS 523 W151t 2006] I. Mitchell,
Robert, 1969– II. Title. III. Series.
RD127.W35 2006
362.17'83—dc22   2005025993